"You're Crazy!"

And other ignorant things doctors have told patients that need brain training

Dr. Kevin Conners

Dr. Kevin Conners has earned his Fellowship in Integrative Cancer Therapy, Board Certified in Integrative Cancer Therapy; Fellowship in Anti-Aging, Regenerative and Functional Medicine, Board Certified in Anti-Aging, Functional and Regenerative Medicine; American Academy of Anti-Aging Medicine; currently studying for Certification in Cardiovascular and for Diplomate Status in Neurology, Carrick Institute as well as the Nutritional Diplomate program; graduated in 1986, Northwestern Health Sciences University though not practicing under such license; Fellowship in Health Research Outcomes, National Institutes of Health; over 100 hours postgraduate study in Autism Spectrum Disorders; practicing Applied Kinesiologist. He is the author of 7 published books including "Stop Fighting Cancer and Start Treating the Cause", and "Help, My Body is Killing Me", and numerous videos available on Amazon. Dr. Conners frequently lectures to doctors around the world at various seminars. Personally, Dr. Conners has been married to his high school sweetheart for over 31 years, has five children and eight grandchildren (and counting).

Dr. Kelly Halderman

Dr. Kelly Halderman is a member of the professional staff at the Upper Room Wellness Center in Vadnais Heights, Minnesota. She practices solely under her Pastoral Medical license, specializing in the care of members with neurological and autoimmune issues using natural therapies approved by the PMA. She is certified by the American Functional Neurology Institute and uses cutting-edge, innovative therapies such as Neurofeedback outlined in this book. She holds presentations on Neurofeedback and lectures all around the country on Lyme disease, as well as a host of other topics such as nutrition and homeopathy. Dr. Halderman has an extensive healthcare background, as she trained in Family Practice with the University of Minnesota Family Medicine Residency program after graduating from traditional medical school in 2007 and is also a graduate of Kingdom College of Natural Health though she does not hold a state medical license nor practice medicine. She also holds a certificate in Plant-based Nutrition from Cornell and is a graduate from the Institute for Integrative Nutrition.

CONTACT US:

Upper Room Wellness Centers, **651.739.1248**

www.drkevinconners.com   www.upperroomwellness.com

If any of you lacks wisdom, let him ask God, who gives generously to all without reproach, and it will be given him.
-James 1:5

Dedications

Years ago I dedicated myself to Christ. Though I often fail, I am reminded over and over that He loves me no matter what. Also, 31 years ago, I dedicated myself to a wonderful woman. Without her love and encouragement I would never be able to accomplish a work like this as she gives me the time to pursue my passion of continual study.

Thank you Terri, I'll always love and cherish you!

There is nothing better than knowing that you are living in the light of His glory and that your eternity is secure, but life this side of heaven can have its share of complications.

Our practice is dedicated to a calling. Our mission, per say, has been and will always be molded around helping others with both life's complications and coming to experience the reality of the love of God and His promises for a future.

Praise God that His mercies are new each and every day!

Forward

Maybe it's just human nature for a doctor to blame the patient when they have no answers; I'm not quite sure. I do know that I've heard dozens of patients tell me that they were 'written off' by their general practitioner and usually told to see a psychiatrist. Personally, I believe the psychiatric field has its place but to dismiss a person with a dis-functioning brain and make them feel like they are lying or worse, crazy, is a shame. I can understand that no one wants to fail and if the patient's symptoms don't fall into the doctor's perfect categories, they just have no idea what to do.

Though we will never claim to have all the answers, our promise has always been to admit our ignorance and devour data to try to find an answer. When I lecture to other doctors I impress upon them the 'drive to finish life' with few regrets. Professionally, it would be sad to complete a career in healthcare knowing that you did anything less than your best to find and solve every patient's problem. I believe that any patient seeking my help was sent by God and it is my responsibility to do my best to 'figure them out'.

Though I've been trained in the alternative healthcare field, I'm the first to admit that sometimes the best thing for the patient is appropriately used medication. Unfortunately, we see far too many individuals seek our care that have had medications that have seemingly been prescribed simply to shut them up. The, "Try this drug," approach has been disguised as the practice of medicine in an age that preaches evidence-based care. Doctors have become technicians following manuals written by pharmaceutical companies. Gone are the Marcus Welbys who used years of accumulated wisdom mixed with modern day common sense. We have strict practice guidelines that keep doctors pawns to higher powers in healthcare that generate revenue for corporations that care little of the individual.

This book is not going to explain everything you need to know about brain-based issues but it is our hope, above everything else, to give you HOPE. There IS a reason you may feel like you're going crazy; there IS an explanation for your memory loss, your focus issues, brain fog, depression and anxiety. Your child's ADD/ADHD is not genetic and not some strange punishment from God. If you never should walk in our door, please find some door where a doctor seeks your best, desires to find the cause and is less apt to blame a label. Always know that God made you and He loves you! Feel free to contact us for help professionally or send us your prayer requests:

www.UpperRoomWellness.com

Upper Room Wellness Center
1654 County Road E E
Vadnais Heights, MN 55110
651-739-1248

"My longings, my hopes, my dreams, and my every effort has been to live for Him who rescued me, to study for Him who gave me this mind, to serve Him who fashioned my will, and to speak for Him who gave me a voice."

— *Ravi Zacharias, Jesus Among Other Gods: The Absolute Claims of the Christian Message*

"You are never too old to set another goal or to dream a new dream."
- C. S. Lewis

Introduction

While I made every attempt to make this book as simple as possible, the brain is a complex organ. I apologize for it becoming a text book at times but honestly, there is just so much to be said and I get so excited about the possibilities. For the general public, some parts of this book are going to be really boring and much too technical. For doctors not educated in functional medicine or functional neurology, it may be insightful and spark a new desire to learn and help the patients no one else can help. For the trained physician, it may be a book to hand out to patients so they may be better able to understand what you are trying to do.

I originally wrote the beginning of this book several years ago with every intention of getting the information out to my patients. But, as is often usual in my life, God had different plans. My practice is primarily to member patients with cancer and severe autoimmune disorders including many that are mentioned in this book so while I have been doing less and less brain-based therapy, completing this book appeared less than necessary. But again, both time and God, change things.

When Dr. Kelly Halderman, an MD trained through the renowned University of Minnesota Medical system entered our office and shared her personal story, her desire to help patients at a deeper level, her frustration with standard pharmaceutical-medical procedures, as well as her love for God and desire to serve Him, we knew it was a fit from heaven. She has taken functional neurology to the next level in our clinic and inspired me, with her help, to complete this work. It may be important to note that because both Dr. Halderman and I seek to use only natural, biblical methods of care supported by the Pastoral Medical Association; neither of us are licensed to practice medicine, chiropractic, or any profession licensed by the state, nor do we wish to do so.

Again, please forgive the textbook feel at different points and understand that this is a work in progress as we will continue, as I have in the past with all my other books, offer them for free online and be updating the downloadable copies as needed.

My deepest desire is that someone is blessed and given new hope by what they read.

Sincerely,

Dr. Kevin Conners

Chapter One

Can Anybody Fix ME?

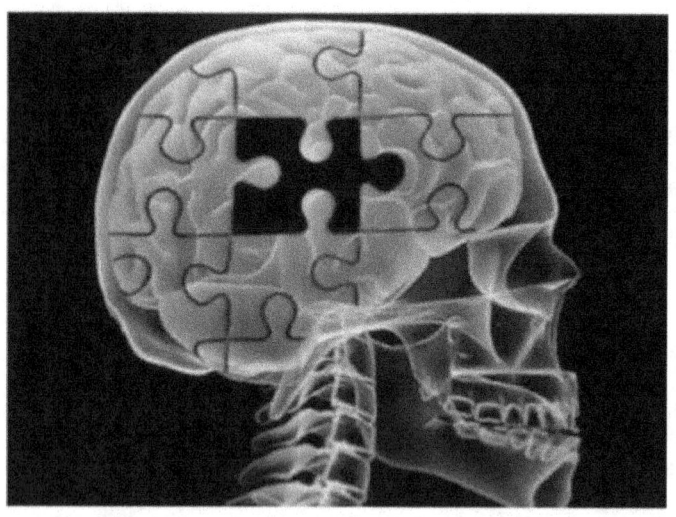

Or am I just CRAZY?

– A model for change for ADD/ADHD, Asperger's, Autism, Anxiety, Depression, Panic, Fear, Anger, Bi-Polar, Chronic Fatigue, Chemical Imbalances, Fetal Alcohol/Drug Syndrome, Dementia, Multiple Sclerosis, Alzheimer's, PTSD, Post Concussive, Chronic Pain, Mood Disorders, Thyroid and other Hormone imbalances, Autoimmune disorders, and more.

Neurobehavioral disorders such as listed above, share many features in common, so many that I and others who treat patients from a neurological and functional medical perspective see them as a spectrum or what I call, a 'circle' of one disorder. Honestly, I am against labeling a patient with a diagnosis; believing that a name given to a collection of symptoms simply forces one to *own* the disability, I think it is wiser to teach the patient to understand 'why' the symptoms are present and help them through the process of correcting the reason they are there.

In the past we referred to such neurobehavioral disorders as Disabilities, Mood Disorders or Chemical Imbalances; currently these terms have fallen the way of both neurological and political incorrectness. Functional Neurologists like to call them 'Disconnection Syndromes'.

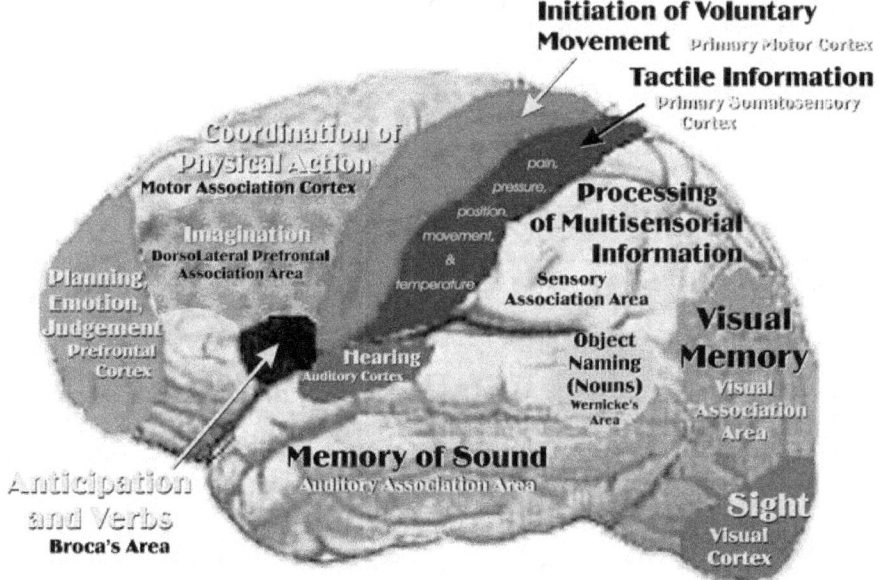

Anxiety, Depression, Panic, Fear, Anger, Bi-Polar, Chronic Fatigue, Chemical Imbalances and Mood Disorders fit directly into the same mold as Attention Deficit Disorder, Attention Deficit Hyperactive Disorder, Pervasive Developmental Disorder, Obsessive-Compulsive Disorder, Asperger's Syndrome, and Autism to name but a few, and may be viewed as points in a 'circle' of Disconnection Syndromes in which those points share features in common. The etiologies or causes of these Disconnection Syndromes share a common bond as well and we might add other brain degenerative conditions to the mix as well such as Alzheimer's, Parkinson's, and the dementias.

Though we give these disorders separate names and ICD (diagnostic) codes to classify them for insurance reimbursement and drug clarification, this book will explore their similarities and the way a functional neurologist may explore the possible solutions.

Though each Disconnection Syndrome may vary as to the part of the brain that is affected, I like to view these disorders as points on a circle:

ADD/ADHD

PDD-NOS   Depression

OCD   Anxiety
                                                      Bi-Polar

Panic Attacks   **Brain**   Paranoia
                         Disconnect

Asperger's   Autism

Addictions   Tourette-like

Dementia   Loss of Empathy
                    Anger issues

Chronic pain, Parkinson's, Alzheimer's, and other issues like post-concussion syndrome fit into this picture as well and understanding the very simple fact that the brain controls everything will help the reader understand.

As the functional medicine and functional neurological community currently understand the developmental disabilities of this circle, let us explore some specific fundamentals that will help you understand how you can be helped should you struggle with any brain imbalance:

1. THERE IS OFTEN AN IMBALANCE BETWEEN THE TWO HEMISPHERES, THE DIFFERENT BRAIN CENTERS, AND/OR THEIR NEURONAL CONNECTIONS. The two halves of the brain are referred to as cerebral and cerebellar hemispheres. These are separated into 'lobes' and 'gyri' with particular and distinct functions. When we are discussing the 'circle' listed above, we are mainly talking about the frontal, temporal, and parietal lobes, and their connections to deeper brain centers. For example, there are common neurological deficits in all the Frontal Lobe disorders even though patients may still present with different symptoms. The primary problem relates to the imbalance between both right and left frontal hemispheres and/or an inability of the frontal lobes to neuronally fire back onto the deeper brain centers that govern autonomic and emotional function.

   Normal (asymptomatic) individuals exhibit an asymmetric distribution of nearly all human functions within the cerebral cortex including cognitive, motor, sensory, neuro-hormonal, immune, autonomic, and endocrine functions, i.e. the left side of the brain controls things that the right does not and visa versa.

Though we now understand that there exists an unbelievable ability of the brain to 'take up the slack' of an underperforming neighbor, it may not exactly jump to volunteer for the extra work.

Neuroplasticity is the buzzword in neurology today and speaks to the brain's ability to remold and reshape to necessary needs, but it often takes a little coaxing. Functional Neurologists like buzzwords; they like big words. Personally, I like words like neuroplasticity because if you break it down it explains exactly how God made us – with the innate ability to adapt to our environment and be molded and shaped for the better.

Brain Based Therapy is a method of shaping and molding. It's the 'little coaxing' we use to re-train the brain around damaged or dysfunctional centers. It's all about balance. Failure to develop and maintain this balance of inter-hemispheric (between sides), inter-lobal (between parts), and inter-glial (speaking of the non-neuronal brain cells we will discuss later) communication or damage affecting such balance between each center results in a form of 'functional independence' that creates havoc. I think it's pretty cool that tiny neurons were created to function in symphony with others, not independently. It is kind of a microcosm of life – we are to be interdependent, interconnected beings, sharing life with others.

Even though the cartoon below is a gross over-simplification of how our brains work, it gives you an understanding in the importance of proper balance. We will see that both developmental issues and, more commonly, environmental issues are most prevalent in causing such imbalances and that such imbalances are never normal and may be the cause of severe emotional upsets.

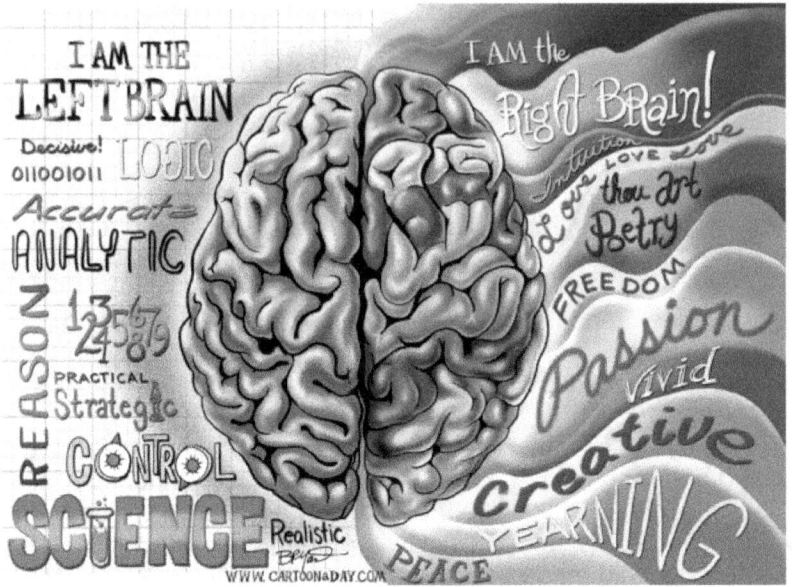

2. MANY CONDITIONS IN THIS CIRCLE OF DISORDERS ARE THE RESULT OF A RIGHT OR LEFT HEMISHPERE DEFICIENCY. Most Frontal Lobe syndromes can clearly be related to dysfunction or delay in development/function of one hemisphere. For example, if the right hemisphere is under-stimulated resulting in slower temporal processing within that hemisphere, it decreases effectiveness of the right hemisphere's normal executive functions. We'll explain more about this later.

In the case of a right hemisphericity (decreased firing of the right frontal lobe), there will be a decrease in activity seen in modern functional imaging of the brain (functional MRI, QEEG) which will show a decreased activity in the right frontal and pre-frontal cortex with an asymmetric distribution of activity in the basal ganglia (part of the midbrain) and cerebellum as these are centers that receive the frontal lobe's output.

This right hemisphericity (right hypo-functioning) is possibly the more common finding and may also explain why young boys are affected more than young girls as seen in the gross imbalance in ADD/ADHD and autistic diagnoses. The frequency ranges from approximately 6 to 1 in ADD to 50 to 1 in high functioning autistic individuals because young male brains are more asymmetrical than young female brains because of hormonal differences.

Male brains are more susceptible to prenatal and postnatal influences; these influences, which are thought to consist of maternal prenatal levels of estrogen, create this left greater than right cortical development characteristic of male brains. Dietary and environmental exposures to estrogens also may contribute to these problems. It has been hypothesized that abnormal decreases in dopamine (a brain neurotransmitter) have a greater negative affect on right frontal cortex function than left due to the asymmetrical distribution of dopamine receptors in the brain (there are more dopamine receptors in the right frontal lobe, hence, more susceptible to losses).

As we age, however, this 'imbalance' changes and the effects of puberty on the female brain swings the pendulum in the opposite direction revealing a much greater incidence of anxiety, depression, etc. in females.

Regardless of statistical incidences, people with brain imbalances suffer not only with the symptoms they express but with the ignorance in the medical community regarding diagnosis and solution. Labels are hurtful, and I hate them. They do absolutely nothing to help the patient and pharmaceutical companies are eager to create new diseases to slap on people's foreheads so they can be loyal customers the rest of their lives. It is both unethical and criminal to make people victims of an imagined diagnosis code instead of searching for a cause so the patient may see real and permanent results.

I refuse to label people so if that's what you're looking for, stop reading this book now, go crawl in a corner and give up. This book is for those willing to stand up and say, "Hey, I'm a person and I deserve a doctor who will help me get to the bottom of this and help me find a solution!"

LEFT BRAIN FUNCTIONS	RIGHT BRAIN FUNCTIONS
Small Picture	Big Picture
Verbal Communication	Nonverbal Communication
Small Muscle Control	Large Muscle Control
Intelligence Quotient	Emotional Quotient
Word Reading	Comprehension
Math Calculations	Math Reasoning
Processing Information	Interpreting Information
Conscious Actions	Unconscious Actions
Positive Emotions	Negative Emotions
Receiving Auditory Input	Interpreting Auditory Input
Linear and Logical Thinking	Gets Abstract Concepts
Curious and Impulsive Actions	Cautious and Safe Actions
Like Routine/Sameness	Likes Newness, Novelty
Activates Immunity	Suppresses Immunity

3. ENVIRONMENTAL INFLUENCES CONTRIBUTE TO THE PROBLEM. Some main factors in causation of frontal lobe disabilities are hypothesized to be

environmental, especially in the more severely afflicted. Current socially acceptable behaviors, primarily those which are sedentary, such as a high proportion of time spent watching television, on the computer or playing video games (all highly left brain stimulants), are at least a factor for the dramatic increase in neurobehavioral problems.

The human brain is extremely plastic (moldable, changeable) allowing us to adapt to the environment in which we live. The window of time for the greatest development is between conception and the age of six; hence, bad parenting at early ages shapes the child for life. Other than healthy, loving environments, motor activities are critical during this time of brain development, particularly in males. A dramatic decrease in early motor activity in children will affect development of gross motor behavior, which is more specific to right hemisphere development, therefore, decreases in early motor activity equals decrease in right brain development. In more sedentary children, the increased use of TV, DVD, computers, iPhones, and video entertainment coupled with working parents, and parental fears for their children, all stimulate left-brain growth and lack of right brain stimulation.

Other environmental factors such as poor nutrition, increased poor caloric intake, environmental toxins, and early sensory deprivation are other important factors which we will discuss in greater detail later and are something that we heavily address in our office. This is the 'functional medicine' (metabolic) piece that is absolutely essential if a patient is going to recover.

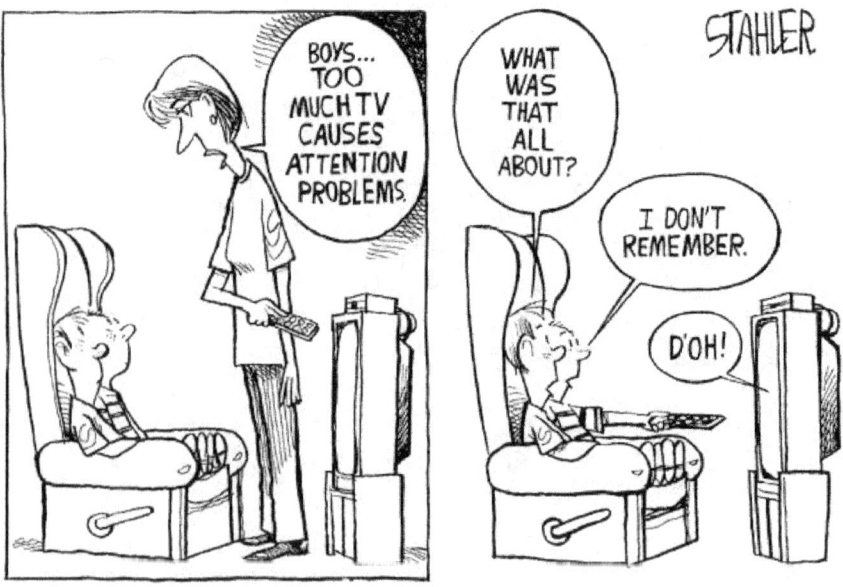

4. DEVELOPMENTAL INFLUENCES CONTRIBUTE TO THE PROBLEM. Though this has become the minority of cases we currently see, every patient has need for revisiting developmental stages. Persistent neurological reflexes that *should* disappear at specific developmental stages can linger to cause problems. We discuss remediating these in later chapters. Years ago I saw more developmental-delay issues due in part to common parenting practices at the time like the use of baby swings, playpens, Johnny Jump-ups, baby walkers, etc. that would restrict necessary cross-crawl activity crucial for brain development. Social and cultural understanding of the detriments of these things has decreased (at least with what we see in our office) the frequency of developmental problems but the sudden rise in inflammatory causes more than offsets any benefits of our efforts in educating parents about detrimental parenting practices during developmental stages.

> *"Rabbit's clever," said Pooh thoughtfully.*
> *"Yes," said Piglet, "Rabbit's clever."*
> *"And he has Brain."*
> *"Yes," said Piglet, "Rabbit has Brain."*
> *There was a long silence.*
> *"I suppose," said Pooh, "that that's why he never understands anything."*
> *— A.A. Milne, Winnie-the-Pooh*

5. INFLAMMATORY INFLUENCES CONTRIBUTE TO THE PROBLEM. We will discuss much about this topic as I cannot recall a single patient in recent history that did not have some source of brain inflammation. Neurological pathways that are blocked or damaged from an immune attack or any source of inflammation simply cannot function properly. Thinking that you will have a healthy brain and be able to eat processed foods, McDonalds French fries, and a Slurpee just reveal that you may already have brain problems. We'll talk about the destructive problems of GMO foods, excitotoxins (additives meant to increase taste and cause food addictions and thereby increase repeat sales), food coloring, preservatives, additives, etc. Also see my book, "Help, My Body is Killing Me…" for more on this topic.

6. TRAUMATIC INFLUENCES CAUSE FUTURE PROBLEMS. The Center for Disease Control (CDC) has now issued major concerns regarding long-term issues of traumatic brain injuries. There is also a huge concern now in the sports world as some data lists an unbelievable discrepancy in adult-onset dysfunction in all brain disorders (Alzheimer's, early Dementia, Parkinson's) with individuals who've played contact sports, especially professional football players. Some studies even reveal a decreased life expectancy! There are functional changes that occur in how the brain works but often no structural damage can be seen on standard imaging tests like CT scan, yet the chronic, sub-clinical inflammation consumes neurons like the heat of a slow burning fire.

Mild traumatic brain injury, or concussion, can be defined as a short-lived loss of brain function due to head trauma that resolves spontaneously but can have lasting ill-effects. The brain floats in cerebrospinal fluid and is encased in the skull. These protections help us to withstand many of the minor injuries that occur in day-to-day life. However, if there is sufficient force to cause the brain to bounce against the skull, then there is potential for injury. It is the acceleration and deceleration of the brain against the inside of the skull that can cause the brain to be irritated and interrupt its function and, more importantly, sets up a chronic inflammatory process that slowly decreases function and destroys neurons.

While temporary loss of consciousness due to injury means that a concussion has taken place, most concussions occur without the patient being knocked out. Studies of football players find that the most of those affected were not aware that they had sustained a head injury. The chronic inflammatory processes that ensue not only destroy neuronal and glial function but bring fibroblasts that create adhesions and rigidity within the brain and between dural layers that cover the brain and spinal cord.

7. ALL OF THESE CONDITIONS ARE VARIATIONS OF THE SAME PROBLEM. Most brain disabilities are of similar etiology and are variations of the same underlying problem. The frontal lobes, temporal lobes, parietal lobes, cerebellum, basal ganglia, and thalamus have been implicated in all of these conditions. This has been documented on static imaging such as CT scans and MRI, as well as functional imaging such as PET scans, QEEG and fMRI. Bottom line: inflammation in the brain blocks pathways that need to be 're-mapped'. The pathways that are damaged equal the symptoms the patient experiences giving a diagnosis specific to those symptoms.

John was a real estate agent in southern California for over 30 years. He was looking forward to semi-retirement and being able to spend more of his time playing golf, which was his passion. A few months ago he noticed a strange sensation, beginning in his legs that was slowly, over time, creeping upward. "It wasn't pain," he described, "it was a weird stiffness; sometimes it was tingly, other times it was achy, but it got worse every day." John never went to a doctor, though he complained to his wife who would demand that he make an appointment. But he was stubborn and, like many men, just pretended it would be better tomorrow. After about 4 months, John's stiffness became so bad that, when at his son's house for a family function, he couldn't get out of a seated position in the couch. That was the final straw that landed John in the ER. I'll save some time and skip over most of John's story and spare you the miserable months that followed with MRIs, CT scans, X-Rays, etc., and these *after* the ER just sent him home with prednisone telling him it was stress.

John was diagnosed with Multiple Sclerosis, early stage, which 'has yet to show plaquing'. This wasn't the end of his story though because John had a dream to retire and play golf and his dream was not going to be side-lined by some crazy disease the "he was going to have to learn to live with". He never gave up asking why and was willing to seek care beyond the confines of multi-million dollar facilities that offered no hope. The 'end of his story' was a beginning in a sense because John end up at a Naturopath's office that had attended a seminar of mine, was referred for a phone consultation. After much consideration, John and his wife flew in for a complete work-up and we all learned new and amazing things. John learned that there was hope (he's nearly completely recovered), I learned that even medications can be antigens in an autoimmune condition (it was Lipitor in his case), and my staff learned that a patient's drive to fulfill a life-long dream can be an essential motivating factor to getting better.

Unfortunately, there are millions of people who do not have the insight to see beyond traditional medicine and believe they 'have to live with' whatever disease they've been told they have. We see it every day. Yesterday, one of my assistants told me about someone at church who was telling her that her son's absence seizures were coming more frequently and that he's had multiple grand mal seizures in the past month. The doctors increased his seizure meds but the meds seem to just, 'wipe him out.' After my assistant attempted to try to explain that there may be hope looking through a Functional Neurology and Functional Medicine lens, the woman interrupted with a, "oh no, they found the 'cause'; they said it's genetic."

People are people. Somehow a 'diagnosis' seems to emotionally erase the responsibility of really figuring things out. If we can just blame a disease or a gene that is outside of our control then we absolve ourselves of any accountability. Yet the suffering continues. I cannot begin to tell you how many cancer victims we speak with every day that have been to hell and back with 'therapies' that have left them mutilated, yet fear, tradition, and peer-pressure pushed them down a medical path that left them crumbled in a corner like a dirty rag.

If the only thing you get out of ANY of my books is HOPE, then I've succeeded! Find someone near you that understands the thing we write about. I teach doctors world-wide and we see patients in our office from around the world yet we are still amazed by the neighbors willing to let their children suffer a lifetime from a 'genetic' brain problem!

8. THESE PROBLEMS ARE CORRECTABLE. Because brain organization is plastic (changeable), many aspects of neurobehavioral disorders do not have to result in permanent impairment (unless left alone). Appropriate forms of "re-mapping" (Brain Based Therapy, Neurofeedback) and behavioral modifications (Neural Cognitive Therapy) can significantly improve or completely correct the underlying problem. Since motor and cognitive

dysfunction often coexist, improving the function of one effect change in the other.

Annie, an eight-year-old beauty with long black hair and princess eyes was a handful. Her parents had three other children, all younger than Annie with two still in diapers. "I'm just worn out," confessed her mother, a thirty-something, dedicated homemaker who was at the end of her rope. "We've tried everything we know," explained her dad, "yesterday the school's counselor had recommended either you or medication, but said we have to do something now." Annie had been on medication last year for the ADHD her pediatrician diagnosed. Like most kids, she did not do well, "It just made her completely groggy," said mom, "she had no personality."

It's always nice to see parents "at the end of the line" because they seem to be more willing to do the hard things that it takes to get their child better. It's kind of like that with all patients; if they aren't sick enough to make drastic life-style changes, then they are NOT going to get better. Not that every case needs dramatic life-style changes but the willingness to do so is crucial. I once had a family with a teen-ager who was in juvenile detention, soon to be in prison that absolutely refused to remove gluten from their diet because, "pizza was his favorite food". Just shoot me now!

Praise God that Annie's parents were committed. They could see beyond immediate gratification to the hope of recovery. Maybe that is the sign of a healthy brain – one who can put-off immediate satisfaction for a future, attainable goal. Annie's a different person today because her parents had a healthy brain. Yes, we needed to change her diet, detox heavy metals and teach her brain-based exercises to do at home and yes, the results were both dramatic and gradual but she is now in high school getting excellent grades.

Functional Neurology and Functional Medicine offer us intervention strategies including Advanced Neurofeedback, home Brain-Based therapy, functional testing, kinesiology, and other labs that can both reveal true, underlining causes and show marked positive effects and objective changes in a relatively short period of time. Using the newer therapies we suggest in this book, most of our patients now notice significant changes in months as opposed to years (or never).

9. HEMISPHERE SPECIFIC TREATMENT AND INFLAMMATORY CAUSE IDENTIFICATION IS THE KEY TO SUCCESS. Besides increasing motor performance, timing, endurance, and posture, we will finally address the need for hemisphere specific treatment modalities. Brain Based Therapy, sensory stimulation, and cognitive functions directed toward the under functioning hemisphere are the most important consideration in treatment. Achieving a balance of activity between the two hemispheres is critical for allowing cognitive and bilateral motor binding to occur, which would reduce

hemispheric neglect (hypofunction). As the hemispheres achieve a normal coherence and synchronization, motor and cognitive performance will improve. Below is the ONLY way that we believe one will achieve lasting results:

A. Determine the specific brain gyrus that is NOT firing correctly. This is done through a detailed neurological examination and a "Brain Map" using a functional electroencephalogram (EEG). Our Neural Integration software system lays out a detailed explanation of improper brain function.

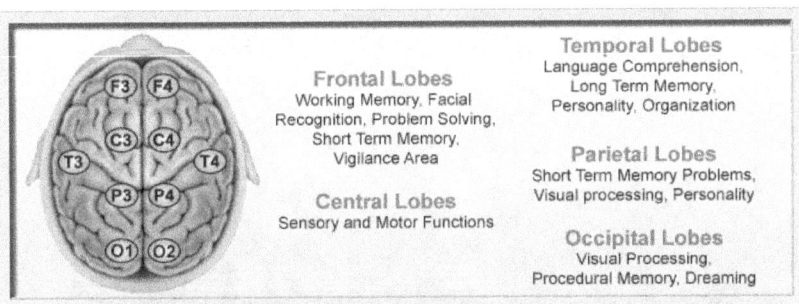

B. Determine the CAUSE. Most common causes are inflammatory processes from toxicity, autoimmune inflammation, or trauma. The patient is experiencing an EFFECT. If they ever expect to recover from the effect, the cause must be discovered and removed.

C. Determine a plan of attack to REMOVE the cause. Treatment is appropriate to the cause.

D. Develop specific Brain-Based Therapies that RE-WIRE the brain pathways that were damaged.

This above approach seems simple, and, though it is working wonders to prove that people are NOT 'crazy', it requires that your doctor or doctors are aptly trained in functional neurology and functional medicine. I certainly don't consider myself an expert as I am always learning (maybe addicted is a better term) but, as the title of this book state, regardless of what your previous doctors have told you, there IS an answer.

There are REAL causes to problems that require solutions not found in a new prescription or another label. It is true that you will not find the therapies we suggest referenced by pharmaceutical companies but NOT true that what we do and suggest for patients doesn't work or has little validation. Functional EEG's (one of our primary therapies) have MORE positive research data and proven clinical trials than any drug on the market! The problem is that there is no money to be made by Big Pharma! I hate to be cynical but it's both sad and true.

For more research, see our site: www.ClearMindMinnesota.com

Chapter Two

What IS Normal?

Normal Brain Function

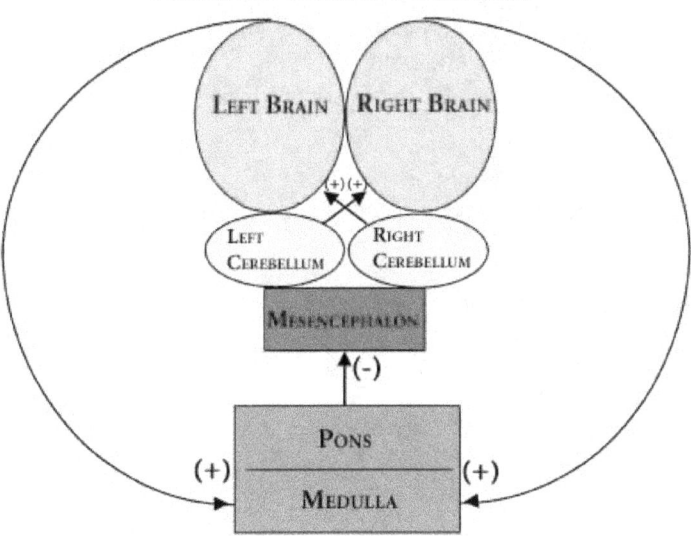

"I didn't want normal until I didn't have it anymore"

— Maggie Stiefvater, *Lament: The Faerie Queen's Deception*

BRAIN FUNCTION OVERVIEW (in general)

Left Brain
- Analytical, judgmental; more in-the-box thinking
- Works with familiar information – anything new/novel fires the right brain first, then it becomes a left brain function
- Language fluency (speaking and reading)
- Broca's and Wiernicki's areas of left temporal lobe
- Math skills that are more linear – 2 + 2; whereas word problems are more right brain
- Enjoying your surroundings
- Processing information from detailed facts
- Repetition and systems
- Happy brain
- Dull/monotone voice
- "What" function ("What shape is this object?")
- Causes action: goes and gets

Right Brain
- Creative and emotional
- Works with new information
- Nonverbal communication (body language and facial expressions)
- Social skills
- Drawing/art
- Reading comprehension
- Humor
- Gross motor skills
- "Where" function
- Causes withdrawal and regeneration
- Rhythmic voice

Temporal Lobe
- Memory (hippocampus): long term = inferior lobe; short term = superior lobe
- Speech
- Verbal communication
- Auditory attentiveness
- Understanding of sound and music

Occipital Lobe
- Vision

Parietal Lobe
- Hand motor control
- Processes sensory information from the environment

Frontal Lobe
- Sense of self, ego, personality
- Ability to focus and not be impulsive (ADD, ADHD)

PMRF (PontoMedullary Reticular Formation)
- Function of cardio-respiratory center
- Maintains global muscle tone and upright posture in gravity

Cerebellum
- Sensory and motor processing station
- Receives input from all other brain regions
- Sends sensory input from the body to all other brain regions
- Determines smoothness of movement and thought
- Maintains tone of spinal muscles
- Posture, balance, coordination

Mesencephalon (upper brain stem)
- It's function is controlled by the other brain areas (frontal, parietal, cerebellum)
- If these areas are fatigued, the mesencephalon overfires, causing—
  Chronic pain
  Migraines
  Racing heart
  Jaw tension
  Irritable bowel
  Insomnia
  Other symptoms often found in chronic conditions

Brain Development

Oh, the sheer excitement of the above title. My neurology professor (30 years ago) was a terrible teacher and I never learned a thing about the brain. It would be decades later that I was introduced to Professor Carrick and life changed. I discovered that human behavior, though governed by choice, is shaped largely by the intricate function of a few pounds of fatty tissue encased in relatively thin bone. It's amazing really; humans who build skyscrapers that touch the clouds, engineer moon landings, cage giant animals ten times their size, and rule the world have not enough bodily hair to keep from freezing to death on a cold night, no claws sufficient for gathering enough food for the day, teeth too small to rip through an animal should carrion be found nor skin thick enough to able to defend even an attack from a large group of mice. No, we were created to use our brains.

Most neurological texts would dive into evolutionary theories on how fish brains lack a neocortex and as we evolved from slime we simply decided to grow neuronal hemispheres capable of reason. It takes at least as much faith to believe that as it does to believe there is a grand weaver who has a sovereign plan. If you want to get technical about it, thousands of years ago, humans had bigger brains. That conclusion was reached after researchers showed that ancient human skulls from Europe, the Middle East and Asia had an average brain capacity of 1500 cubic centimeters, compared to today's 1359 cc.

> "I consider that a man's brain originally is like a little empty attic, and you have to stock it with such furniture as you choose. A fool takes in all the lumber of every sort that he comes across, so that the knowledge which might be useful to him gets crowded out, or at best is jumbled up with a lot of other things, so that he has a difficulty in laying his hands upon it. Now the skillful workman is very careful indeed as to what he takes into his brain-attic. He will have nothing but the tools which may help him in doing his work, but of these he has a large assortment, and all in the most perfect order. It is a mistake to think that that little room has elastic walls and can distend to any extent. Depend upon it there comes a time when for every addition of knowledge you forget something that you knew before. It is of the highest importance, therefore, not to have useless facts elbowing out the useful ones."
> — Arthur Conan Doyle, A Study in Scarlet

The old skulls tested were almost certainly post-Flood, hence at most a few thousand years old by biblical reckoning, and 'only' tens of thousands of years old in evolutionary belief. If the result had shown that today's brains are bigger, this would no doubt have been interpreted by evolutionists as humans evolving more 'smarts'. But this outcome has caused a quiet surprise—not just for being contrary to evolutionary expectations, but because of the extent and speed of change. John Hawks of the University of Michigan called it "a major downsize in an evolutionary eye-blink". That said, I will do my best to make this section readable and keep you from falling asleep because even though the facts may be 'dry', understanding them explains much about problem behavior.

Over the centuries scientists have argued two dominate views on human development. They proposed that children either came into the world genetically pre-programmed ("nature") or that they were a "blank slate" on which their environment shaped their development ("nurture"). Lately, the debate over nature vs. nurture is fading as scientists now are investigating the complex ways in which genes and environment interact in part due to the completion of the human genome project that exposed the failure of the 'genetically preconditioned' camp. It turns out that we have fewer genes than expected – far fewer! It is 'genetics' that we can blame all our problems on, it's 'epigenetics' (what our environment does to affect the genes). Current brain science understands that both nature and nurture shape brain development, and that each set of influences is dominant to varying degrees at various points in time.

Before birth, nature is the primary actor in brain development. We certainly cannot dismiss the effect of environment as any parent of a Fetal Alcohol Syndrome child would attest, but the pre-programmed genetic map runs the show at this stage. According to Dr. Pasco Rakic, a professor of neuroscience at Yale University, "The number of neurons and the way that they are organized is determined by heredity." We know that during the third week of pregnancy, a thin layer of cells in the developing embryo folds inward to create a fluid-filled cylinder called the neural tube. (Berk, 1994, p. 99). It is in the neural tube where the production of neurons, the brain cells that store and transmit information, begins at the rate of 250,000 per minute (Nash, 1997, p. 52). Here is where environmental toxicity may interrupt genetic processes.

By the end of the second trimester, the process of producing neurons is essentially completed. It was once believed that no more neurons would ever be produced again in an individual's lifetime – a topic now hotly debated. Some neurons are programmed for specific functions such as breathing, controlling the heartbeat, regulating body temperatures, or producing reflexes – all depending on the pathways on which they are created. But, for the most part, neurons are not designated to perform specific tasks, and thus brain development is not complete at this point. Think of neurons as highways on which communication travels.

Brain development is "stimulus-dependent," meaning that the electrical activity in every circuit—sensory, motor, emotional, and cognitive--shapes the way that circuit gets wired. Similar to computer circuits, neural circuits process information through the flow of energy (electricity). Unlike computer circuits, however, the circuits in our brains are not fixed structures. Every experience--whether it is seeing one's first rainbow, riding a bicycle, reading a book, sharing a joke--excites certain neural circuits and leaves others inactive. Those that are consistently turned on over time will be strengthened, while those that are rarely excited may be dropped away. This is neuroplasticity and it is both good and bad. If my first experience with the world was an inattentive parent who neglected me, I may experience adult behavioral issues with getting needs met. We neurologically tie connections to feelings, experiences, events, object identification, color, sound, and every conceivable stimulus.

What functional neurologists say, "Cells that fire together, wire together," meaning connections are made, not hard-wired. The elimination of unused neural circuits, also referred to as "pruning," may sound harsh, but it is generally a good thing. It streamlines children's neural processing; making the remaining circuits work more quickly and efficiently. Without synaptic pruning, children wouldn't be able to walk, talk, or even see properly. But it goes both ways. If a two-year-old is never taught social behavior skills, pathways of 'normal' behavior far outreach cultural acceptance. Also, abused or neglected children create pathways of worthlessness that become superhighways easily traveled throughout life. This is the neural connection to "sins of the father carrying out to the third and fourth generation." The cycle must be broken.

At any stage of development, other environmental toxins including maternal malnutrition, substance abuse (including alcohol, smoking, illegal drugs, and use of prescription and over-the-counter medications), exposure to chemicals or radiation, vaccinations, pathogens (like Lyme and other bacteria) and viral infections (such as measles) can lead to adverse effects on the developing brain. It goes without saying then that even the most loving parents; living in the fallen world which is inescapable with its chemical, EMFs, and destroyed food supplies (GMOs, additives, pesticides, herbicides...) can have children with brain issues. It's NOT about blame; it's about recognition and correction!

While newborns are born with a full set of neurons, the most important part of brain development begins after birth - the wiring phase. Following birth, each of the brain's 100 billion neurons creates links to thousands of others (Nash, 1997, p. 53). This process is accomplished as neurons produce a web of wire-like fibers called axons (which transmit signals) and dendrites (which receive signals). Once axons make their first connections, the nerves begin to fire (Nash, 1997, p. 53). It is at this point that the environment begins to take over in the process of brain development. Scientists often describe this stage as the equivalent of creating telephone trunk lines between the right neighborhoods in the right cities. At this point in development, the brain has to sort out which wires belong to which house (Nash, 1997, p. 53). It is with these maps that learning will take place (Carnegie, 1994).

The most important factor in this process of developing connections is stimulation, or repeated experience. Scientists now know that in the months after birth the number of synapses increases from 50 trillion to 1,000 trillion (Carnegie, 1994). Neurons that are stimulated by input from the surrounding environment continue to establish new synapses. Those that are seldom stimulated soon die off.

According to Dr. Harry Chugani, a professor of pediatric neurology at Wayne State University, .It's like a highway system. Roads with the most traffic get widened. The ones that are rarely used fall into disrepair. (Nash, 1997, p. 26).

It's not black and white, it's GREY and WHITE

The nervous system is divided into components based on location: the central nervous system and the peripheral nervous system; as well as function: the volitional system and the autonomic system. Then there are other divisions; the autonomic is divided into the sympathetic and parasympathetic based on opposing functions. The central nervous system is composed of the brain and the spinal cord. The brain is then divided wholly into grey and white matter. Scientists are very left-brained and enjoy memorizing systems and names and big words that make you sound really smart.

Grey matter (say substantia grisea – it's Latin for grey matter and makes you feel like you know what you're talking about when you say it), is the part of the brain that is made up of nerve cell bodies and the majority of the true dendrites (numerous, short, branching filaments that carry impulses towards the cell body). Grey matter has no myelin blanket; it is simply the collection of cell bodies.

The real processing is conducted in the grey matter. It was given the name gray because, wait for it – it's grey. Neurons create networks, in which nerve signals travel and though we speak of connections, they do not make contact with each other when conveying messages, but do so through sending chemicals across a gap called a synapse. The chemicals called neurotransmitters serve as the medium to connect one neuron to another neuron. The senses of the body (speech, hearing, feelings, seeing and memory) and control of the muscles, are part of the grey matter's function.

> *"But when you're in front of an audience and you make them laugh at a new idea, you're guiding the whole being for the moment. No one is ever more him/herself than when they really laugh. Their defenses are down. It's very Zen-like, that moment. They are completely open, completely themselves when that message hits the brain and the laugh begins. That's when new ideas can be implanted. If a new idea slips in at that moment, it has a chance to grow."*
> — George Carlin, Last Words

The white matter, also known as substantia alba (no, not Jessica Alba's daughter though that would have been my first pick), is a neuron that is made up of extending, myelinated nerve fibers, or axons. It composes the structures at the center of the brain, like the thalamus and the hypothalamus. It is found between the brainstem and the cerebellum, between the neocortex (newer brain centers) and lower brain. It is the white matter that allows communication to and from grey matter (nerve cell) areas. It functions by transmitting the information from the different parts of the body towards the cerebral cortex; the white matter is the axons. It also controls the functions that the body is unaware of, like temperature, blood pressure and the heart rate. Dispensing of hormones and the control of food, as well as the intake of water and the exposition of emotions, are additional functions of the white matter. Communication along these fibers reaches a speed of 2-300 miles per hour (remember this for the quiz).

Because of the evidence emerging on synaptic development, scientists believe that appropriate stimulation of the child's brain is critically important during periods in which the formation of synapses is at its peak (Berk, 1994). It is during these critical periods, or windows of opportunity that exist for different brain functions, when a child's experiences can make the most difference. And, for some areas, if the connections between neurons are not developed during these critical periods, they will never develop at all.

Nutrition is so important in every stage but crucial in the early years. The average Western diet has changed dramatically such that humans today consume a much higher proportion of omega-6 fatty acids relative to omega-3 fatty acids than ever before. The importance of omega-3 fatty acids in human development has been well established in fetal and neonatal development, with brain and retinal tissues highly dependent on omega-3 fatty acids, specifically docosahexaenoic acid (DHA) for membrane fluidity and signal transduction. In childhood, omega-3s have been shown to contribute to ongoing cognitive development so supplementation with DHA is highly recommended. (Carlson, 2013)

This is why I've always said that a fat-free diet is the most dangerous diet known to man. Did you know that there is a phenomenon known as rabbit starvation? Yes, it is described by observing settlers that ate nothing more than rabbits, which were in abundance, and filled their bellies, yet died of starvation. The lack of fat in rabbit meat (tastes like chicken) was the killer. You NEED fat; pregnant mothers and children need fat even more (eat coconut oil). There, now you can't say that you didn't learn a thing from this book!

One area of brain development that has received much attention in determining its critical period is vision. It has been found that the synapses associated with vision multiply quickly in 2- to 4-montholds and keep increasing until around 8 months (Jabs, 1996, p. 25). At 8 months, each neuron is connected to 15,000 other neurons (Begley, 1996, p. 56). This rate makes sense when we realize that infants have limited motor skills and spend much waking time watching the world around them. Yet researchers have found that a baby whose eyes are clouded by cataracts from birth will, despite cataract removal surgery at the age of 2, be forever blind. This finding indicates that the window of opportunity for vision does not stay open for a long period of time.

Other deficiencies have been well established as to the detrimental effects on the brain but a recent rat study revealed that EMF exposure from cellphones significantly damages cells in the brain. "Widespread use of mobile phones which are a major source of electromagnetic fields might affect living organisms," the study states. "Two groups of pregnant rats, a control group and an experimental group that were exposed to an electromagnetic field were used. For obtaining electromagnetic field offspring, the pregnant rats were exposed to 900 megahertz electromagnetic fields during the 1–19th gestation days. There were no actions performed on the control group during the same period. It was found that 900 megahertz (typical cellphone EMF) of electromagnetic field *significantly reduced* the total pyramidal cell number (the area of brain dissected) in the brains of the rats exposed to the electromagnetic field. (O Bas)

Fetal alcohol syndromes (FAS) as well as fetal drug exposure are conditions that result from alcohol and drug exposure during pregnancy. Problems that may be caused by exposing the developing brain to such chemicals include physical deformities, mental retardation, learning disorders, vision difficulties and behavioral problems. The problems vary from child to child, but defects caused by chemicals can sometimes be irreversible as brain centers can completely be obliterated. There is no amount of drug (even OTC), tobacco, alcohol, vaccination that's *known* to be safe to consume during pregnancy. If you drink during pregnancy, you place your baby at risk of fetal alcohol syndrome. (Mayo)

Does this research mean that it ever becomes too late to make a difference in the brain development? Bite your tongue! God made us plastic, moldable, changeable, so even damage done at early, important stages can, with proper assistance, change and re-mold. Researchers have found that the brain during the first years of life is very malleable, citing instances in which very young children who suffer strokes or injuries that wipe out an entire brain hemisphere still mature into highly functioning adults (Nash, 1997, p. 54). Children have also been found to overcome emotional and physical abuse suffered during the first year, presumably because of plasticity, or the ability to rewire damaged brain areas.

It is also important for parents not to push children during this period and provide too much stimulation. This is why I'm against attempting to make your child a prodigy with Baby Einstein-type educational toys that over-stimulate the left frontal lobe. Parents who try to rush children through the necessary stages of development are asking children to function with capacities that may not be ready to be used (Jabs, 1996, p. 25). In addition, if parents try to push children, they may form connections between certain activities and stress. Parents who try to force a child to complete a puzzle before he or she is developmentally ready may decrease the child's disposition to do the puzzle or engage in related activities because of the stress connection.

With few exceptions, (vision as perhaps one notable exception) the windows of opportunity in brain development do not close abruptly. What research findings do indicate are the importance of helping children develop a sound foundation in early learning, so that they have the building blocks for a lifetime of learning.

A study published in tomorrow's issue of the journal *Science* shows that social interaction during a critical period of early life has irreversible effects on maturation of connections to the frontal lobes of the brain, disrupting social interactions and cognitive ability into adulthood. Children suffering severe neglect are known to have cognitive dysfunctions and impairments in social interaction as adults, but the mechanisms were not understood.

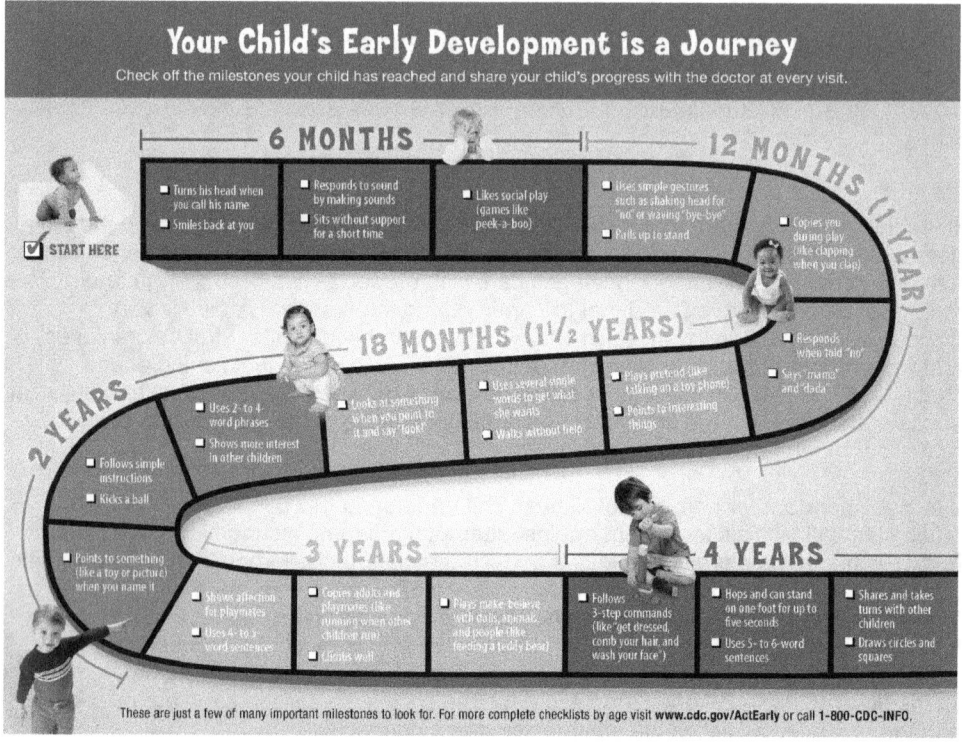

Your Child's Early Development is a Journey

Check off the milestones your child has reached and share your child's progress with the doctor at every visit.

These are just a few of many important milestones to look for. For more complete checklists by age visit **www.cdc.gov/ActEarly** or call **1-800-CDC-INFO**.

Situated behind the forehead, the prefrontal cortex is responsible for complex analysis, abstract thought, motivation, and controlling socially correct behaviors. Interestingly, connections from other brain regions to the prefrontal cortex are not fully developed until the early twenties.

There has long been speculation as to the development of behaviors attributed to frontal lobe functioning in children. Problem behaviors attributed to frontal lobe dysfunction are evident yet controversies as to whether it is because of ill-development or a lesion (damage due to trauma, toxins, inflammation) continue to arise. (Passler) .A team led by neurobiologist Gabriel Corfas at the Children's Hospital in Boston reared mice in isolated cages for two weeks after they were weaned from their mothers. When these animals reached adulthood, the nerve fibers (axons) connecting to the prefrontal cortex had a thinner coating of electrical insulation (myelin) than in mice reared in standard cages (in community, with their mothers).

Myelin insulation, wrapped around axons like electrical tape, greatly increases the transmission speed of nerve impulses. Slower transmission of information to the frontal cortex could degrade performance of this critical brain region. Indeed, behavioral experiments showed that these animals had poor working memory and impaired social interaction as adults.

Real world: Anything that causes a decrease in firing of cortical centers leads to dysfunction! This includes developmental delays due to everything from nutrition to lack of love. But this is important – we are NOT just talking about children! Every second of your life your brain requires stimulation; if you don't use it, you lose it. Period; exclamation point. Poor use of grammar I know, but I want you to get his point.

"Mice are normally interactive socially and tend to be gregarious and investigative, and in some cases also aggressive among themselves, but these mice [reared in isolation] tend to avoid interacting with animals that are placed into their same cage," Corfas says. It is all because of poor formation of prefrontal connections. It is well documented that disruptions in social interactions in humans are associated with many psychiatric disorders. Worse, the researchers found that reintroducing mice into a normal social environment after the two-week period of isolation did not restore normal myelination or improve performance on tests of memory and social behavior as adults. Moreover, social isolation later in life did not have the same effects as social isolation immediately after weaning. It takes much more brain-training to recover what is lost in 'critical periods' of development.

This shows that there is a sensitive period in early life when social interactions are necessary for normal myelination of axons to the prefrontal cortex. "The findings make sense and are consistent with what we've observed in clinical studies on effects of early stress on the brain," says Martin Teicher, a neuroscientist in the Department of Psychiatry at Harvard University.

Using MRI brain imaging, Teicher and his colleagues have found that early life stresses, including childhood sexual abuse, witnessing domestic violence, and experiencing verbal abuse from parents or peers, affect the structure of the prefrontal cortex and disrupt fiber connections to this and other brain regions. Many alterations in brain tissue could produce the differences seen by MRI in children suffering neglect, but by removing the tissue and examining it under an electron microscope, Corfas and colleagues were able to prove that indeed myelin was thinner on these axons in socially isolated mice. "This is the first study to show that it is enough to change myelin to produce the behavioral effects that you would expect to be caused by isolation," Corfas says.

The Prefrontal Cortex

In order to explain this important part of your brain that sits directly in back of your forehead I need to tell you about the Disney movie UP, Adolph Hitler, a Roman General, and my dog Lady. For those of you who have not seen Pixar's UP, you now have some homework because the humorous observation of the dogs in this animated blockbuster give real insight into the prefrontal cortex.

In the story, balloon salesman Carl Fredricksen and his energetic wife Ellie live a wonderful life with dreams of adventure that always seems beyond financial reach. After Ellie's death, Carl grows quiet and confined until meeting 8-year-old Wilderness Explorer Russell who is eager to get his "helping the elderly" pin. Without retelling the entire story, this unlikely duo travel to a faraway land and meet the antagonist as well as new friends like Dug, a dog with a special collar that allows him to speak, and Kevin, a rare 13-foot tall flightless bird (but a very nice bird, as all Kevin's are).

Before you start thinking that I have ulterior motives for having children, there is a great lesson in the story's antagonist's (famed explorer/inventor Charles Muntz) dogs. Fitted with their talking collars, the dogs pursue the pair to capture their new friend, the exotic bird Kevin. In doing so we see the truth about dogs – they have a very small prefrontal cortex, as I'm sure you were thinking as well when you watched the movie.

Once, when capture seemed inevitable and the adventure doomed to failure as the talking dogs were at the verge of victory, Russell ingeniously distracted the animals from their goal by shouting, "Squirrel!" The prefrontal cortex is necessary to stay on task, remain focused on intention and block out distractive issues. Humans should have no problem with focus, dogs do. No matter how obedient to their evil master the dogs desired to be, dog are dogs and dogs chase squirrels.

The prefrontal cortex intention; it is the the students on task would be chaos directly lesion. It is primarily allows attention on schoolmaster keeping and without it there proportional to the responsible for regulating behavior, mediating conflicting thoughts, making choices between right and wrong, and predicting the probable outcomes of actions or events. It governs social control, such as suppressing emotional or sexual urges. Since the prefrontal cortex is the brain center responsible for receiving data from the world and deciding on actions, it is most strongly implicated in human qualities like consciousness, general intelligence, and personality. It is what makes us unique as humans – the size of our prefrontal cortex.

> *"Every man can, if he so desires,*
> *become the sculptor of his own brain"*
> *— Santiago Ramón y Cajal*

It was the summer of 1941, the plan was simple, but Hitler was alone in his thinking that it would be simple to perform. Given the size of Russia, the German army would be divided into 3 groups. Army Group North would advance through the Baltic States towards Leningrad, Army Group South would move into the Ukraine and then the Caucasus to take the wheat and oil fields of Russia, and Army Group Center would advance through White Russia towards Moscow.

Germany had already conquered most of Europe and the Fuhrer's success following his planned Blitzkrieg was unprecedented. He thought Germany was unbeatable and he trusted his track record over wise counsel. This obstinacy became the cause of many heated debates between Hitler and his Generals and proved disastrous for "Operation Barbarossa," the attack on Russia. When a country goes to war, it is only sensible that the Government and the Military have already determined the enemy's "Center of Gravity", and have already planned on how to neutralize it. The enemy's "Center of Gravity" can be their armed forces, their capital, a powerful ally, etc.

Hitler and his Generals disagreed from the start about what Russia's "Center of Gravity" was. The Generals thought it was Moscow, while Hitler thought it was Ukraine and the Oil fields of the Caucasus. Hitler's reasoning, if it can be called that, was based on history. Napoleon had taken Moscow, but the Russians had not given in, and in the end Napoleon had to retreat, with disastrous results for his Empire. Hitler was determined not to repeat that mistake; he was going to head south, take the Ukraine and the Oil fields, and deny the Russians the resources he felt they needed to continue the war.

His Generals could not have disagreed more. They argued that Russia was so vast, and capable of replacing whole armies, that only the capture of Moscow would destroy the Soviet Regime. They argued that Moscow was the political and logistical hub of European Russia, and if it was taken, the Russians would not be able to continue the war west of the Urals. A simple glance at any world atlas will indeed show that in Western Russia, "all roads lead to Moscow."

The General's reasoning was that since most of Russia's population, resources and industry were located west of the Urals, even if the Russians elected to fight on, it would be a lost cause. Finally, they argued that Stalin was so feared and despised, (nearly a million citizens took up arms against Russia's military) that if the Red Army was destroyed, and Moscow taken, the people would overthrow him and welcome Germany's rule.

Hitler was a ruthless dictator, and therefore had the last word; in this case he was absolutely wrong. The attempt to seize of Ukraine in 1941 was blind optimism, born out of pride in the heart of a deranged tyrant. Even if the Germans had taken Ukraine and all of the oilfields, the Soviet Regime would still be intact and worse, given the still considerable Russian armies to the north and the long lines of communications the Germans would have in the south, the Russians could have possibly cut off the German army in southern Russia as they actually did in late 1942.

What does this have to do with the prefrontal cortex? Recent research on why we do what we do has concentrated on decision making. There appears to be a dichotomy in cognitive neuroscience between reflective versus reflexive decision making. Reflective, goal-oriented, or what has been termed model-based thinking is now been shown to be a right prefrontal function. This means if I have greater left-brain dominance, I will be more prone to habitual, less reasoned, or what is known as model-free decisions. Right-brain dominant people base decisions more on perspective thought, weighing consequences, and seeing possible outcomes. Left-brain dominant individuals make choices more on what was done in the past, patterns that are common, and "the way I've always done it." It goes without saying that evil dictators have brain problems but I think most have two severe (very severe) lesions: right dorsolateral and right anterior cingulate damage.

A study published in Neuron in October, 2013 showed that disrupting the right dorsolateral prefrontal cortex impaired flexible model-based choices, driving behavior toward simpler, model-free (habitual) control. Blind pride may have more of a neurobiological cause than previously believed. Damage to prefrontal brain structures has been documented in psychopathic criminals as well.

These studies show that human choice behavior often reflects a competition between inflexible computationally efficient control (from the left brain) and a slower more flexible system based on weighing factors and consequences (the right brain) on the other. One can see that BOTH are necessary for optimal performance in a complex world. A commander of armed forces, a CEO of a major company and a parent of small children need healthy functioning frontal lobes to both make quick decisions based on past experience and slower, more carefully thought out choices based upon reason.

There are times we all need reflexive, non-emotional decision-making that will be efficient and give us a good chance that the outcome will be similar to past outcomes based on similar circumstances and there are other times where being able to imagine all sides of either ruling will guide us to the best selection. Imbalance is not healthy.

Would World War II have had a different outcome had Hitler had a more balanced brain? Well, yes, it wouldn't ever have started had Hitler had a healthy prefrontal cortex. We could write an entire book on his traumatic childhood, his mother's death of cancer, and his brain problems and conditioning but it suffices to say that one could explain all ill-behavior, no matter if demonic or innocent as having at least part of its origin in the prefrontal cortex.

Here's something really cool for you nerds out there. Recent research on why we do what we do has concentrated on decision making. There appears to be a dichotomy in cognitive neuroscience between reflective versus reflexive decision making. Reflective, goal-oriented, or what has been termed 'model-based' thinking has now been shown to be predominantly a right prefrontal function (versus the left prefrontal). This means that if I have greater left-brain dominance, I will be more prone to habitual, less reasoned, or what is known as 'model-free' decisions.

Right-brain dominant people base decisions more on perspective thought, weighing consequences, and seeing possible outcomes. Left-brain dominant individuals make choices more on what was done in the past, patterns that are common, and "the way I've always done it."

A study published in Neuron in October, 2013 showed that disrupting the right dorsolateral prefrontal cortex impaired flexible model-based choices, driving behavior toward simpler, model-free (habitual) control.

This and other studies show that human choice behavior often reflects a competition between inflexible, computationally, efficient control (from the left brain) and a slower more flexible system based on weighing factors and consequences (the right brain). One can see that BOTH are necessary for optimal performance in a complex world.

"What is human memory?" *Manning asked. He gazed at the air as he spoke, as if lecturing an invisible audience - as perhaps he was. "It certainly is not a passive recording mechanism, like a digital disc or a tape. It is more like a story-telling machine. Sensory information is broken down into shards of perception, which are broken down again to be stored as memory fragments. And at night, as the body rests, these fragments are brought out from storage, reassembled and replayed. Each run-through etches them deeper into the brain's neural structure. And each time a memory is rehearsed or recalled it is elaborated. We may add a little, lose a little, tinker with the logic, fill in sections that have faded, perhaps even conflate disparate events.*

"In extreme cases, we refer to this as confabulation. The brain creates and recreates the past, producing, in the end, a version of events that may bear little resemblance to what actually occurred. To first order, I believe it's true to say that everything I remember is false." — Arthur C. Clarke

There are times we need reflexive, non-emotional decision-making that will be efficient and give us a good chance that the result will be similar to past outcomes based on similar circumstances and there are other times where being able to imagine all side of either ruling will guide us to the best selection. Imbalance is not healthy.

Mirror Neurons

My dog Lady is a great friend. She's obedient (for the most part) and since she's aged a few years, she's just the level of mellow that I like in a pet. She drives me crazy though when I'm busy doing something like carrying groceries from the car or running to the barn to get the power drill. Wanting my immediate attention, I find myself frustrated with her uncanny ability to position herself exactly in the direction I'm moving. "Look out Lady," I cry, as she moves again precisely where I was planning to step. She has absolutely no sense of self! She has no idea that she's 'in the way' because she doesn't even know that she is she. She cannot possibly see my point of view, cannot place herself in my situation, and cannot understand my intention because she has no sense of being.

What makes humans human? We are born completely dependent on mom and take years to develop; but Lady was wrestling with her brothers just minutes after her birth. Brett, my first grandson, took months to roll over, longer to sit up on his own and nearly a year before he walked and finally blurted out what was deep inside him since birth, "Grandpa is my favorite." Lady on the other hand seemed to possess near her current intelligence weeks after birth and though her fondness for stealing shoes has diminished, she's been Lady as I know her now since she was a pup.

Humans are different. We are more neurologically advanced yet it takes years, even decades, to mature through stages that lower species seem to conquer in days or weeks. Why? It seems rather counterintuitive. Shouldn't higher level species have evolved a quicker defense against predators and be able to progress more rapidly to higher consciousness? Let's talk about a special class of brain cells called mirror neurons.

We humans learn much of what we know by imitation. As neurons myelinate, our sense of self becomes keen and soon we are able to do something lower species cannot – we can adopt another's point of view. The ability to see the world from another's point of view is a complex function that my dog will never possess. Her frontal lobe is too small! I might embarrassingly add that often my frontal lobe acts as if it is equally small when I fail to see things from her point of view and blurt out expletives that I later regret.

The ability to create a mental model of another's complex thoughts, called theory of mind, is unique to humans. Though Disney makes movies where animals reason and plan and argue and contemplate and set goals and give advice, Lady and her fellow non-homosapiens, no matter how many times I may say, "Can't you SEE I'm carrying groceries," will never understand. It's tied to our ability to converse; our language to convey to another what we think about, how we feel, and even how we feel they feel about us. I can understand a complex dramatic plot and enjoy watching The Notebook because I possess mirror neurons (I've never actually watched The Notebook). I know what you're thinking – I've finally solved the age-old quandary and can now explain it to men everywhere: women have more mirror neurons! This may actually be true, but we'll discuss this another time.

Mirror neurons enable you to simply watch someone do something and fire the same brain circuit as if you did the same thing. They enable you to imagine doing something and fire the same circuit as if you actually did it. This is why I get an unpleasant sensation course my body when I watch Funniest Home Videos and see a skateboarder miss a rail and why I get a chill up my spine when I hear a patient explain how they missed the last step before tumbling to the tile. I have mirror neurons. Watch someone get pricked with a needle and you'll fire pain pathways that can be measured on EEG scans.

It's amazing really. We have the unique ability to empathize intimately with another's misfortunes. We have the exclusive skill to learn, strategize, and contemplate what others may be contemplating. Humans can wonder. Mirror neurons give us the capability to blur the boundary between self and others.

I've asked patients, "If I stepped on your foot, where would you feel the pain?" They, of course answer, "my foot." "Really," I play. "The receptors for pain may be in your foot but you actually experience the pain in your parietal lobe, on the opposite side. It is the neuronal cell body in the primary sensory cortex in the parietal lobe that feels the pain and that then sends messages to the frontal lobe to make decisions about and react to such a stimulus."

The ability to even contemplate the above paragraph required receptors in your auditory cortex to send messages to the frontal lobe and so on. Why am I boring you with this mental yoga? Because it's extremely important when we are talking about problems that people have that would possess them to read a book like this. Mirror neurons are in the brain and problems in the brain cause problems with mirror neurons.

Depression, in part, can be explained as the inability to inhibit the mirror neuron pathway perseverating on impending doom; anxiety is the inability to inhibit fight or flight centers. Autism and Asperger's is an obvious fracture of mirror neurons revealing countless symptoms of one's inability to see anything beyond the narrow tunnel of immediate gratification. They are chained, like Lady, to whatever degree of inability to see beyond their current point of view.

A healthy 'free will' is only possessed by those with healthy cortical mirror neurons. We can consciously inhibit most motor functions and 'override' mimicking another's behavior but autonomic function still prevails. If I tell my daughter there is a spider on her back, she'll scream, sweat, panic, jump and throw her hands up in that girl-ish way girls do even before proving my assertation with hard evidence. That was her 'learned' response (I never taught her that, it must have been her mother). She fired real pathways.

> *"The neural processes underlying that which we call creativity have nothing to do with rationality. That is to say, if we look at how the brain generates creativity, we will see that it is not a rational process at all; creativity is not born out of reasoning."*
> — *Rodolfo R. Llinás, I of the Vortex: From Neurons to Self*

As we will see in later chapters, the ability to control these pathways is health. Phobias are over-firing learned circuits; OCD, tics, PTSD, and panic attacks are the same – inability to control mirror neuron circuits. The same is true for someone stuck in self-pity, narcissistic personalities, and violent criminals with no hesitation to harm another. Healthy individuals can inhibit circuits that less healthy people can't and the fact that inhibitory pathways can be strengthened is the very reason we wrote this book and gives hope to civilization!

The Limbic System

Limbic is an odd Latin term meaning the edge or border. It's where we get the word "limbo". It's an intermediate state between two important places. Early anatomists saw this area of the brain, that which is between the important neocortex and the midbrain as the 'in-between area', or limbic lobe. The limbic system includes one of the following on each side: the hippocampus, amygdala, and other named structures in the temporal lobes that we won't be discussing. (Some experts would also include parts of the hypothalamus, thalamus, midbrain reticular formation, and olfactory areas in the limbic system.)

Are you bored yet? Hang in there as you may spot some relevance as we discuss symptoms when these structures aren't working well. The Limbic System houses several important structures to anyone with behavioral or emotional issues.

First let's discuss the hippocampus because it has such a groovy name. Historically, the earliest hypothesis was that the hippocampus was involved in the sense of smell. Now we know that it is more tied to memories of different smells and how a particular smell of let's say German potato salad instantly connects us to Grandma's house on Thanksgiving when you were 5. Over the years, anatomists have whittled down several main ideas of hippocampal function: inhibition, memory, special order, and circadian rhythm.

The behavioral inhibition theory (caricatured by O'Keefe and Nadel as "slam on the brakes!") was very popular up to the 1960s. It derived much of its justification from two observations: first, that animals with hippocampal damage tend to be hyperactive; second, that animals with hippocampal damage often have difficulty learning to inhibit responses that they have previously been taught.

The second major theory relates the hippocampus to memory. This idea stems from a famous report by Scoville and Brenda Milner describing the results of surgical destruction of the hippocampus (in an attempt to relieve epileptic seizures), in a patient named Henry Gustav Molaison, known until his death in 2008 as H.M. The unexpected outcome of H.M.'s surgery was a specific type of amnesia: H.M. was unable to form new memories after his surgery and could not remember any events that occurred just before his surgery. He retained memories for things that happened years earlier, such as his childhood. This case produced such enormous interest that H.M. reportedly became the most intensively studied medical subject in neurological history.

There were then other patients with similar levels of hippocampal damage and amnesia (caused by accident or disease) have been studied as well. There is now almost universal agreement that the hippocampus plays some sort of important role in memory and most agree its role is more similar to the part of the brain that the original anatomists placed it than they could ever imagine because it is a 'check station' for working memory (things happening now) to pass through to long-term storage (in the temporal lobe).

What does this mean to you? Well, if you've ever walked into a room and asked yourself that stupid question, "What did I come in here to get?" then you've experienced a "blip" in your hippocampus. Working memory, or current thoughts and plans, needs to shunt back from the planning centers in the prefrontal cortex, through the hippocampus to the temporal lobe where they are stored for future use. "Honey, will you get me the scissors in the kitchen," spoken when I'm in the middle of writing a section on the limbic system ends up with me standing in the kitchen with absolutely NO idea of why I was there. In this case, brain chatter caused incomplete processing of frontal lobe commands.

Is it just age that brings about a greater incidence of "senior moments"? If so, then somebody tell me why my teenager can't seem to follow simple instructions even if I tattooed them on her arm. Yes, chatter, disinterest, and not really paying attention will cause working memory issues but abnormal attention problems and continually forgetting where you placed your keys or having to depend more on lists than ever before are all signs of hippocampal damage, most commonly caused by inflammation. We'll talk more about causes in a later chapter but right now, let's just admit we may have a problem.

The third important theory of hippocampal function relates the hippocampus to space. The spatial theory was championed by a very influential book, "The Hippocampus as a Cognitive Map". As with the memory theory, there is now almost universal agreement that spatial coding plays an important role in hippocampal function. A cognitive map is a type of mental representation (you could say your 'mind's eye') which serves an individual to acquire, sort, store, recall, and decode information about the relative locations (where) and attributes (what) of phenomena in their everyday spatial environment.

You could say that the hippocampus works to sort experiences into respective files and then recover them for future use like a file clerk carefully labeling those little plastic tabs that go on the green hanging files and systematically placing all the important papers in the perfect alphabetical order. Boy, am I dating myself! Maybe a better example would be how I acted just like a hippocampus this morning when I sorted all my Word documents into neat files on my desktop so I wouldn't have to spend 45 minutes trying to find a handout on liver/gallbladder flush to give to a patient (like I did yesterday).

> *Some people feel guilty about their anxieties and regard them as a defect of faith but they are afflictions, not sins.*
> *-CS Lewis*

Some researchers view the hippocampus as part of a larger medial temporal lobe memory system responsible for general declarative memory (memories that can be explicitly verbalized—these would include, for example, memory for facts in addition to episodic memory). Damage to the hippocampus does not affect some types of memory, such as the ability to learn new motor or cognitive skills (playing a musical instrument, or solving certain types of puzzles, for example). This fact suggests that such abilities depend on different types of memory (procedural memory) and different brain regions.

Finally we'll discuss the hippocampus' role in circadian rhythm, you know, that smooth Jazz band that your Uncle Larry listens to. No, the circadian rhythm is the cyclical output of hormone release. This timekeeping system, or biological "clock," allows us to anticipate and prepare for the changes in the physical environment that are associated with day and night, energy needs of the body and brain, and sleep patterns thereby ensuring we will "do the right thing" at the right time of the day.

When I hear patients say things like, "I can't fall asleep", or "I fall asleep fine but then wake and can't get back to sleep," I think, "They have a screwed-up hippocampus" (or sometimes I think, "I'd really like a peanut butter sandwich" – but let's not confuse things here).

Cutting through all my ridiculous attempts to bring my really stupid humor to a rather boring topic, let's review some things about the hippocampus before moving on:

- It may be important in behavioral inhibition along with the prefrontal cortex
- It is very important in shunting working memory to long-term storage
- It is important in sorting and retrieving memories
- It may tie memories of special senses (smell) to events, people, or places
- It helps with hormone output as it connects to the hypothalamus and pituitary gland
- It may help tie emotional memories to the amygdala as we shall soon see
- And, it's a fun word to say

Next we'll discuss the amygdala. It sits at the end of the hippocampus, on both sides of the brain and I thinks it's the name of a French, cream-filled pastry. Its central nucleus produces autonomic (non-conscious) components of emotion (e.g., changes in heart rate, blood pressure, and respiration) as well as conscious perception of emotion primarily through the prefrontal cortex (anterior cingulate cortex, orbitofrontal cortex, and dorsolateral prefrontal cortex). Important to note is that these pathways go both ways which controls emotional behavior, fears, and anxiety.

The amygdalae perform primary roles in the formation and storage of memories associated with emotional events. Research indicates that, during fear conditioning, sensory stimuli reach the amygdalae, particularly the lateral nuclei, where they form associations with memories of the stimuli, especially if there is a strong emotional connection. Memories of emotional experiences imprinted in reactions of synapses in the amygdala elicit fear behavior. Fear behavior may be described as what you'd experience if a grizzly bear tore your tent door off. Think of that for a bit and then I don't need to describe the loss of digestive control, raw emotions surfacing, sweating, lump-in-stomach, loss of sexual desire, etc.

This technically happens through connections with a grouping of neurons in what's called the central nucleus of the amygdalae and the bed nuclei of the stria terminalis (BNST). The central nuclei are involved in the genesis of many fear responses, including freezing (immobility), tachycardia (rapid heartbeat), increased respiration, and stress-hormone release. This is because it fires directly into the sympathetic nervous system (the flight, fight, or freeze system). So, stimulation of the amygdala causes intense emotion, such as aggression or fear.

An example of a strong stimulation of the amygdala would be a panic attack. Panic attacks are brief spontaneously recurrent episodes of terror that generate a sense of impending disaster without a clearly identifiable cause. PET scans have shown an increase in blood flow to the hippocampus, beginning with the right hippocampus (think right brain – more emotional) and then to the amygdala. Similar but attenuated blood flow increases occurs during anxiety attacks and prolonged stress.

Destructive lesions of the amygdala cause tameness in animals, and a placid calmness in humans characterized as a flatness of affect – no personality. Lesions of the amygdala can occur as a result of Urbach-Wiethe disease where calcium is deposited in the amygdala. If this disease occurs early in life then these patients with bilateral amygdalar lesions cannot discriminate emotion in facial expressions, but their ability to identify faces remains (the anatomical area for face recognition and memory is in the temporal cortex). This is a good example of how emotion in one area (amygdala) is linked with perception in another area (temporal lobe) to create an intense emotionally charged memory.

Any lesions of the amygdala or from the prefrontal cortex connections to the amygdala were shown to be primarily responsible for 'flatness of affect'. This work eventually led to the psychosurgical technique of prefrontal lobotomies (my aunt had this done in the 1930's and lived as a personality-less 'vegetable' for another 60 years). Remember the movie with Jack Nicholson, "One Flew over the Cuckoo's Nest?" The prefrontal cortex sends inputs into the amygdala and severing this input obliterates the conscious connections to emotions, social behavior, and interaction leaving a flatness of affect directly proportional to the size of the lesion.

Likewise, the opposite is true with excitation – lack of inhibition, excessive motive, OCD-like behavior, excessively emotional, etc. Lesions may increase or decrease function of any particular area or its connections to or from such lobe. Remember, by 'lesion' we mean any interference, stimulation or abnormal function.

The amygdala combines many different somatosensory and visceral inputs—this is where you get your "gut reaction". The link between prefrontal cortex (conscious awareness and decision-making), hypothalamus (hormonal response), and amygdala (emotional memory), likely gives us our gut feelings, those subjective yet protective feelings about what is good and what is bad.

One intriguing observation in ASD is the apparent enlargement of the amygdala. The concept of "allostatic overload" (McEwen 2004, and McEwen & Lasley, 2003) was coined hypothesizing a possible biological defect causing an overgrowth. The enlargement of the amygdala would explain an increased activity of amygdalar function in many individuals – a heightened level of fear and anxiety, chronic stress of an 'overly sympathetic' (by sympathetic I am referring to the sympathetic nervous system controlling fight or flight responses) state, and generalized avoidance of social situations.

The amygdala has dense neuronal connections to the visual centers, modulating many levels of visual stimulation. Such visual processing of faces is essential to brain development in the newborn. A child impaired with a lesion in amygdalar connections may fail to fire impulses and lay pathways to the right prefrontal cortex in particular, further leading to social behavior issues as the child ages.

The ventral (front) of the mesencephalon (Midbrain) makes dopamine, a neurotransmitter for the brain. This dopamine projects to a multitude of areas aiding many functions including the cortex for activation as well as the neostriatum. Think of the neostriatum as the "gateway" to the basal ganglia effecting both the direct pathway (which facilitates movement) as well as the indirect pathway (which defacilitates) movement. Long story short – losses in dopamine make the person slow and rigid, both muscular (as seen in Parkinson's disease) and mental (as seen in the dementias).

The neostriatum is composed of three groups of neural structures: the putamen, the caudate and the nucleus accumbens. The putamen relays connections for movement of the peripheral. For instance, if you have lost dopamine to this area, you get the slow, rigid, masking, hypokinetic tremor in Parkinson's disease. If you get too much dopamine to the putamen your arms will fling as in ballismus or chorea.

The caudate, instead of getting dopamine from the substantia nigra in the ventral mesencephalon, gets dopamine from the ventral tegmentum, AKA "mesolimbic area". This area is turned-on by basic emotions. So, when dopamine from this area goes up, your caudate will fire and create motion not to the limbs like the putamen, but rather the face and muscles related to emotions, like eyebrows, lips, cheek muscles and so forth. This is why one cannot help but express facial expressions when experiencing emotions and trained experts, like police investigators, can tell if someone is telling the truth by reading their face. Your facial expressions go beyond volitional control.

The nucleus accumbens is the third portion of the neostriatum. It takes all "positive and euphoric" projections and tells the brain via direct pathway how awesome the experience was. In addiction, for instance, if someone takes one 'hit' of meth amphetamines, it will alter the amount of dopamine to the nucleus accumbens for the rest of their life. On a healthy note, the nucleus accumbens has an important role in pleasure including laughter, reward, and reinforcement learning, as well as fear, aggression, impulsivity, addiction, and the placebo effect. Yes, one can actually decide that they 'like' something and increase dopamine stores in the nucleus accumbens giving us some insight into optimistic personalities!

When someone has emotional, hyperkinetic disorders as in anxiety, insomnia, tics, OCD, ADHD or just poor behavior, the astute clinician should consider an autoimmune response to neostriatal tissue. Numerous research studies have proven that neostriatal antibodies, secondary to autoimmunity is second only to cerebellar antibodies in commonality. Continued firing of these limbic pathways creates neuronal highways, per say, and reinforces the problem.

It's an interconnection, less like a subway map than the lines on a jigsaw puzzle. Yes, neuronal connections are more linear and defined, but what we'll soon see is that neurons also communicate in ways we never dreamed of – through the glial cells that we once thought of as neural glue.

Brain Glue

The brilliant physician, innovator, and professor, Rudolph Virchow was 59 years old when he entered politics, serving in the German Reichstag (1880–1893), while also directing the Pathological Institute in Berlin. He helped shape healthcare reforms introduced in Germany during the administration of Otto von Bismarck. His prolific writings, while mainly on topics of pathology, included many essays and addresses on social medicine and public health.

Virchow's greatest accomplishment was his observation that a 'whole' organism does not get sick—only certain cells or groups of cells. He believed (in medicine) that health opposition to modern came from healthy cells and changing cellular biology and searching for 'cause' was the best practice of medicine. But remember, most doctors believed this concept that today makes doctors like us "quacks"; this was pre-pharma days. In 1855, at the age of 34, he published his now famous precept "omnis cellula e cellula" ("every cell stems from another cell"). With this approach Virchow propelled the field of cellular pathology. He stated that all diseases involve changes in normal cells, that is, all pathology ultimately is cellular pathology.

> *"Great spirits have always encountered violent opposition from mediocre minds.*
> *-Albert Einstein*

He was so openly (and verbally) opposed to Bismarck's excessive military budget that the angered Bismarck challenged Virchow to a duel, a popular way to settle a dispute in the 1800's. Virchow, being entitled to choose the weapons, chose 2 pork sausages: a cooked sausage for himself and an uncooked one, loaded with *Trichinella* larvae, for Bismarck. He was my kind of guy; maybe I should challenge the state boards to the same dual! Bismarck, the Iron Chancellor, declined the proposition as too risky.

It is Virchow who is credited to discovering the special cells in the brain that were once thought to simply 'hold the neurons together'. Hence, neuroglia or glial cells (brain glue) were aptly named and henceforth, ill-studied as they were thought to do little but what their name implied. As we shall see, current research has proven that God truly doesn't make junk and there is little waste in the natural function of cells. Glia have a multitude of functions and many brain problems stem from issues with glia.

Glial cells functions include providing support for the brain, assisting in nervous system repair and maintenance, assisting in the development of the nervous system, provide metabolic functions for neurons, they house the immune system for the brain, provide the barrier from blood-borne invasion, are what make up myelin for quicker neuron pathways and even conduct communications across to adjoining neurons.

There are several types of glial cells present in the nervous system of humans:

Astrocytes are found in the brain's capillaries and form the blood-brain barrier that restricts what substances can enter the brain. These star-shaped glial cells provide physical support to neurons and clean up debris within the brain. They also provide some of the chemicals needed for proper functioning and help control the chemical composition of fluid surrounding neurons, bathing them in nutrition by receiving glucose from capillaries, breaking the glucose down into lactate (the chemical produced during the first step of glucose metabolism), and then releasing the lactate into the extra cellular fluid surrounding the neurons. The neurons receive the lactate from the extra cellular fluid and transport it to their mitochondria to use it for energy. In this process astrocytes store a small amount of glycogen, which stays on reserve for times when the metabolic rate of neurons in the area is especially high. Remember, neurons require two things to stay alive: fuel and activation. Glucose, supplied by astrocytes, is the fuel!

In order to provide physical support for neurons astrocytes also form matrixes that keep neurons in place. In addition, this matrix serves to isolate synapses. This limits the dispersion of transmitter substances released by terminal buttons; thus aiding in the smooth transmission of neural messages. Think of astrocytes as the 'Secret Service agents' of the neuron.

Astrocytes are also garbage collectors, performing a process known as phagocytosis. Phagocytosis occurs when an astrocyte contacts a piece of neural debris with its processes (arm of the astrocyte) and then pushes itself against the debris eventually engulfing and digesting it.

Finally 'coming clean' with acknowledging the long-term risks of traumatic brain injury in American football players, studies for sideline concussion diagnosis and testing for neurological deficits has revealed more startling news. While concussions have been recognized as causes for a spectrum of neurological problems, the consequences of sub-concussive events (repeated trauma without ever being labeled as a concussion) are now being revealed. We are finding that head trauma, whether severe (concussive) or recurrent microtraumas, disrupts the blood-brain barrier (BBB) and the accompanying surge of a specific protein released by the astrocytes (protein S100B) in blood may cause an immune response associated with production of auto-antibodies (antibodies created against self-tissue).

These are super important findings because both patients and doctors have questioned my long-held hypothesis that the BBB is often the real culprit in brain-based disorders. Once the BBB disruption occurs, anything circulating in the blood can enter the CNS and become a source of inflammation. This is the CAUSE of so many problems! The BBB is no longer a protective moat that keeps chemicals, heavy metals, proteins, inflammatory cytokines from a cold or flu, and anything else that happens to be in the blood due to that individual's current state.

This bears summarizing: When repeated traumas occur, studies show, as stated above, that the astrocytes that make up the blood-brain barrier release S100B, a protein that can create an immune response against the astrocytes themselves. Understand the gravity of this. Repeated traumas and concussive events increase the likelihood of the patient developing an autoimmune disorder that destroys the blood-brain barrier!

Other damage to the BBB occurs with every assault listed in this book (toxicities, food additives/flavorings, gluten, alcohol, stress, GMOs, excitotoxins, artificial sweeteners, chemicals, etc.) and everyone, regardless of current symptoms, should be doing things to heal their BBB. Obviously, the first step is to remove the insult. Also, there are several nutrients that are known to help heal the BBB.

Acetyl-L-Carnitine (ALC) protects the blood brain barrier by preserving its integrity on a cellular level. Studies show that a decline in mitochondrial function contributes to the aging process, also carnitine concentration in tissue declines with age. By supplementing your Acetyl-L-Carnitine levels (100mg-1g per day) you can heal the problem at its source and reduce mitochondrial decay substantially.

Research published in the Journal of Neuroscience suggests the chemical sulforaphane, which is found in broccoli and other cruciferous vegetables (cauliflower, cabbage, cress, bok choy, and broccoli), could help boost the condition of the blood-brain barrier if it is damaged.

Activation of the redox-sensitive transcription factor nuclear factor erythroid 2-related factor 2 (Nrf2) plays a pivotal role in the cellular defense against oxidative stress and aides in neuroprotection. Cytoprotective enzymes found in foods listed above also stimulate Nrf2. Curcumin, Green Tree Extract, Alpha Lipoic Acid, N-Acetyl Cysteine Phosphatidylcholine, Vinpocetine, Feverfew extract, Butcher's Broom extract, Ginkgo extract, Cayenne Pepper, Baicalin (from skullcap root extract), Resveratrol, some of the Medicinal Mushrooms, and Coenzyme Q10 are also beneficial.

Microglia are extremely small glial cells that remove cellular waste and protect against microorganisms. Traditionally, microglia are thought to be sedentary in the healthy brain and activate only during episodes of brain injury or disease (such Alzheimer's disease, Multiple Sclerosis and epilepsy), where they play both neuro-protective and neuro-degenerative roles. That thought has changed with recent studies showing that even when quiescent, microglia are highly dynamic and their processes are constantly surveying brain tissue for signs of neural damage. If astrocytes are the Secret Service, microglia are the CIA/FBI.

A role for microglia in normal brain processes, such as plasticity (brain molding) has now been described. Recent data indicate that microglia are able to sculpt developing neural circuits by engulfing synapses and contributing to synaptic pruning. They are resident macrophages (immune system killer cells) of the central nervous system that display high functional similarities to other tissue macrophages that help create and maintain an intact tissue homeostasis to support the neuronal cells, which are very sensitive even to minor changes in their environment.

Microglial cells are the dominant antigen presenting cells in the brain which means they are mainly responsible for keeping infections out of your cranium. Upon attack, they are highly up-regulated and are essential for interacting with T lymphocytes to kill pathogens. This up-regulation is a blessing when the immune system is able to kill an invader but is also a curse if the pathogen is unable to be located leading to an autoimmune disorder such as Multiple Sclerosis. See the section on autoimmune disease later in this book or my book, "Help, My Body is Killing Me..." available on Amazon or as a free download to our website www.UpperRoomWellness.com.

In the case of microglial cells attacking self-tissue in Multiple Sclerosis, they phagocytose (eat away at) myelin (the protective covering of the neurons), degrade it and present peptides of the myelin proteins as antigens to the Th1 macrophages. By releasing cytokines such as CCl2 and Th17, microglial cells are important for recruiting leucocytes into the central nervous system. Microglia interact with infiltrating T lymphocytes and mediate the immune response in the brain. They have the capacity to stimulate proliferation of both TH1 and TH2 responses and therefore are active in all autoimmune brain disorders like Chronic Lyme, MS, ALS, etc.

Calming microglial and therefore calming immune up-regulation is essential in controlling all inflammatory processes in the brain!

Oligodendrocytes produce the myelin sheath, the insulating material that surrounds nerve fibers (axons). This sheath greatly increases the speed at which electrical signals are transmitted, a crucial feature. Learning is greatly dependent on myelination; the very reason that a 4-year old can be expected to act like a 4-year old and not a 2-year old nor a 12-year old is because of the degree of myelination. There is no possible way a newborn can do things that a one year old can; they have few myelinated fibers! Therefore, in an autoimmune reaction as described in the above paragraph, microglia are partially responsible for destroying oligodendrocytes.

All white matter tracts contain oligodendrocytes to form myelin but oligodendrocytes are also found in gray matter. These 'satellite' oligodendrocytes have so far unknown functions possibly serving to regulate ionic homeostasis similarly to astrocytes.

Schwann cells are last type of glial cell and are the cellular counterparts to oligodendrocytes in the peripheral nervous system (outside of the brain and spinal cord), forming the myelin sheath there.

For your Doctor about Healing the BBB

The blood-brain barrier (BBB) is what is often damaged in patients needing brain therapy. The truth is, everyone probably has some damage to their BBB. In attempting to help heal it, I think that we need to understand some vascular biology.

How does BBB damage begin?

It starts in the vessels, both cranial and systemic. Just like heart disease, brain inflammation begins as an endothelial problem. The endothelium is the lining of the arteries and since we are talking about the blood-brain barrier, we'll discuss the vessels that feed the brain. Remember, neuronal function is dependent on both fuel and activation and the fuel is delivered through the arteriole system guarded closely in the brain by the special glial cells called astrocytes.

The endothelium is a single layer of cells that act as a wall with thousands of little gates called receptors that allow certain chemicals in to affect the smooth muscle layer beneath it. If this protective wall gets damaged or the gates get stuck open, we are going to have a problem and a problem in the vessel wall soon spells a problem in the barrier.

Blood testing that should always be considered (and seldom is) with all brain-based symptoms includes a complete vascular profile but measuring cholesterol, HDL and LDL is insufficient in testing out vessel health. All HDL isn't "good" and all LDL isn't "bad." Ask your doctor for more specific tests like *hsCRP*, *Homocysteine*, *oxidizedLDL*, *Lipoprotein A*, and *Apolipoproteine A*.

Your vessels are lined with a single-cell layer of tissue called endothelium; under this endothelial layer is a smooth muscle layer that is responsible for contracting (raising blood pressure in times of needed blood flow) and relaxation (lowering and normalizing arterial pressure in the brain). This endothelial lining is really the KEY; it is the barrier, the wall that allows both willingly and not, changes in the muscle tone as well as invasions into the delicate space underneath.

Let's say this again but start at the beginning. We eat food and impurities hit the first barrier, the stomach. Here, the pH is extremely acidic for two main reasons: it digests (breaking for into smaller particles) and kills pathogens. This second purpose of HCl (stomach acid) is of vital importance as it is the first line of defense against potential destroyers of other barriers like the blood-brain barrier. Helicobacter pylori, for example, are ubiquitous bacteria that should be easily killed by a normal acid balance in the stomach. If you have an imbalanced HCl supply, H. pylori infiltrates and can either cause a stomach or duodenal ulcer or will pass through attacking other organs. It is estimated that 95% of H. pylori infections are chronic, insidious and subclinical – meaning it is rarely diagnosed as a disorder itself and usually the culprit of many other named diseases. H. pylori is such a common cause of vessel damage that leads to both heart disease and blood-brain barrier disruption that I've devoted an entire section on it later in this book.

The second barrier an ingested item encounters is the intestinal wall. Here, cells lining the hair-like villi protect unwanted guests from entering. Proteins, for example, are broken into individual amino acids that are small enough to traverse the cellular barricade. Much of the problem with food sensitivities comes in when separation of the intestinal cells allows food proteins to pass into the blood before they are completely digested into amino acids. These proteins and protein particles called peptides are foreign to the body, stimulate an immune response and our body makes antibodies against them. This is how gluten becomes an autoimmune antigen and wreaks havoc through the body. Again, it all starts with a broken barrier.

The next barrier needing to be crossed is the intimal lining of the blood vessel. Blood flows through the lumen of the vessels and interacts with receptors in the inner covering called intimal endothelial cells. These are barrier cells that allow nutrients to pass to feed cells. All cardiovascular disease as well as every brain disorder discussed in this book starts with endothelial disease! Again, think of the endothelial cell layer as a fence with hundreds of gates called receptors. These gates are opened with specific chemical keys that change the function of the smooth muscle layer behind the fence and can even change the shape of the fence itself. Under normal conditions, chemicals released by tissues knock on the gates looking for permission to enter. For instance, a sympathetic nervous system response (fight or flight) in the brain to a perceived stress causes the release of a chemical that will enter a gate in the endothelial fence to cause the smooth muscle layer to contract and narrow the lumen of the vessel. This increases the speed of blood flow and increases the blood pressure so you can run away from the danger. It is a normal response, but like any normal response, we can get 'stuck' in an 'on' position from chronic source of stimulation.

There are really an endless number of possible insults that could 'breach the gates' of the endothelial wall. Chemical toxicity, heavy metal toxicity, food additives, flavorings, colorings, infections, and endotoxins are just a few of the things that can break the gates and cause damage to the endothelial layer, the small, smooth muscles and tissue underneath, and interact with the astrocytes that act as the next (and special) barrier in the brain. You may have heard about the damage that Homocysteine, glucose, or oxidized LDL cause, but by far, the worst culprit for damage is infection.

Subclinical (silent) infections are the number one 'bad guy' causing endothelial disease which leads to blood-brain barrier disruption. "Subclinical" means the patient doesn't know they have it! It's a silent disorder that can cause mild, insidious vasculature damage for years (and yes, it can start at birth) until the victim has symptoms of ADHD, anxiety, depression, memory loss and dementia, just to name a few. I know this is a lot of info so I'll sum this up:

1. BBB disruption really starts with damage to the endothelial layer – the single-celled barrier that lines the vessels.
2. If the endothelial layer is 'breached', several bad things occur that lead to inflammation in the vessel wall, the tiny muscles underneath the wall, and the astrocyte cells that are meant to keep larger molecules of things out of the CNS
3. Many possible sources of endothelial damage exist due to poor diet, environmental exposure to toxins, and ubiquitous infectious organisms but subclinical infections (unknown to the patient) are the most common and least diagnosed cause of endothelial disease and hence, brain disorders.

Endothelial disease is always the start of BBB disruption and usually never addressed by the any doctor. Heck, most doctors don't even address the fact that there is a disruption in the BBB. Worse, many doctors are still blaming the patient's depression on a chemical imbalance as if it was a disease that poor victim contracted when they were caught out in the rain without a jacket. Medications can change a person's mood, they can numb symptoms, and dull hyperactivity. Medications cannot cure because they do nothing for 'cause'.

Three Possible Responses

There are three possible responses that occur when vascular endothelium is damaged by the infinite number of possible insults:

- a local inflammatory response,

- an oxidative stress response,

- or an autoimmune reaction.

All three possible responses include inflammation, which is the more damaging aspect of each response. Like every tissue, the endothelium maintains a fine balance between injury and repair. It's like a teeter-totter that tips gently back and forth; vessels are damaged by endless assaults and then healed by a collection of innate physiologic responses that viewed as a whole, over time, we call health. If an individual has the unfortunate event of continual and prolonged damage, the repair can actually bring about problems that we shall soon see.

The first response is acute, local inflammation. Let's use an example of vascular injury from high Homocysteine levels. Homocysteine is a toxic byproduct of protein catabolism that is an intermediate metabolite; which means it is supposed to be converted to another nontoxic substance and under normal circumstances it should never accumulate to levels that would injure the body. Homocysteine is highly corrosive to endothelial tissue and sets up a series of events that increase inflammation under the cell lining; it also damages the kidneys as well increasing what is known as the Renin-Angiotensin-Aldosterone-System (RAAS). This RAAS response does several things, including increasing Sympathetic nervous system activity (which increases blood pressure, increasing anxiety, decreasing detoxification…), increases water retention, increases cortisol release from the adrenal glands, increases vasoconstriction, which all work together in your body's attempt to solve the problem of toxic exposure. However, prolonged injury, as in chronically elevated Homocysteine levels, will lead to endothelial disease and BBB disruption (as well as cardiovascular disease).

The second possible response of the vessel is a reaction to oxidative stress, which is an increased production of reactive oxygen species (ROS) and reactive nitrogen species (RNS) – free radicals that can cause severe cellular damage. As I stated, all three reactions cause inflammation and several chemical changes including a down-regulation of the nitric oxide system. Epithelial nitric oxide production is extremely protective to the cell; decreased production of nitric oxide will cycle-up the inflammation in and under the endothelial cell layer.

The third response is the most damaging and is therefore the most dangerous cause of ALL BBB disruption problems – Autoimmune Endothelial Disease (AED). AED is a new term we'll use for an autoimmune reaction occurring in the endothelial tissue. If you've read my book, "Help, My Body is Killing Me…" you will be up to snuff on what an autoimmune disorder is, but I'll review:

An autoimmune disease is a normal reaction of your immune system to a foreign invader that it either cannot kill or isn't killable. Normally your immune system 'turns on' to an enemy attack (bacteria, virus…) and kills it. Should your initial immune response not be sufficient to kill the **antigen** (that which it 'turned on' against) it will gradually increase intensity. The initial 'killer response' is from the Th1 side of your immune response, which might be described as the SWAT team that does one thing and does it well: kill things. Should the Th1 response NOT be able to kill the pathogen, it will suppress, thus allowing the Th2 response to fire. The Th2 response is primarily responsible for making antibodies that 'tag' the antigen so the Th1 killer cells can find and destroy the enemy.

The above is a brief summary of a normal immune response. What can go wrong is if the immune response erroneously turns on against something it shouldn't have – such as heavy metal toxicity, an environmental poison, or some other non-living substance the patient was exposed to. Secondly, the immune system can turn on against something that just doesn't die so easily. Common biotoxins (living organisms that can attack the body) that infiltrate endothelial tissue include: H. Pylori, Coxsackie virus, Chlamydia Pneumonia, Lyme, Cytomegalovirus, Gingivitis, Candida, Strep and Staph.

All these little buggers can burrow into the endothelial cells and create an immune response. Since they have a special ability to go intra-cellular (hide inside the cell), the Th1 response has a difficult time finding them.

Over time, a ramped-up immune response does two things:

1. It destroys endothelial tissue (both receptors and entire cells) due to collateral damage in its attempts to kill the antigen, and

2. It starts to mistake self-tissue for the enemy and begins direct destruction of self-tissue, and

3. An immune response can destroy the astrocyte barrier further allowing antigens to enter the CNS and further the inflammatory spread!

A continual, low-grade immune response as seen in AED and BBB destruction is very inflammatory and usually vasoconstrictive. We'll go into more detail about this and give a various examples to 'drive it home'.

This exact same process can/does occur in the vessels in the brain which causes TIAs and Strokes!

A Common Cause – a case study

Remember that there are three responses of the endothelial tissue: acute inflammation, oxidative stress, and autoimmune disease. Remember that we discussed that the single-cell layer that lines the vascular structures acts as a barrier or wall that has hundreds of gates called receptors that allow interaction between the external world (inside the blood vessel) and the internal world (inside the endothelial cell and then under it).

John was 54 years old and went in for his annual check-up. After a thorough exam and blood work his doctor determined that John's cholesterol, a 203, needed attention. He was also concerned that the slightly elevated blood pressure required medicating and re-assured John that both the Lipitor for his cholesterol and the blood pressure medication at the small dose he was recommending was absolutely necessary to keep John from an early myocardial event like that experienced by John's father.

But let's look at what was really happening: Deep inside John's blood vessels the endothelial layer we've detailed has been infiltrated years ago by foreign invaders. Helicobacter Pylori, an enemy that is more commonly known for causing stomach ulcers is perhaps the most common pathogen to crawl past the stomach lining and invade deeper tissue. H. Pylori bacteria have slowly spread into cells in John's lungs and vessels. Normally an invasion like this would stimulate an all-out attack by local law-enforcement officers (the immune system) but every troop dispersed has found little success as the enemy is cunning and has the ability to enter and hide within the cells it attacks.

Over time, John's immune system has placed H. Pylori on its top ten most wanted list and has waged a silent war against this elusive enemy, often finding it in different areas in the body. The attacks on the H. Pylori found in the endothelium has caused slow, insidious inflammation in the vessels that has opened gates for chemical responses that increased smooth muscle tone under the vascular wall – this is what caused the increase in John's blood pressure.

But John's doctor hasn't bothered to address the cause of John's high blood pressure; he's just prescribed ACE inhibitors to manipulate the numbers. As far as giving him Lipitor for cholesterol levels of less than 400 – well will save that for another time. But it gets worse:

John leaves the doctor's office feeling that he has just added years to his life by artificially manipulating lab values back into a pre-determined range. Far be it from the truth! The CAUSE of John's problem has just continued and the H. Pylori bacteria continue to take a foot-hold in various places including the endothelial layer in vessels around the heart, the lungs and the CNS. Years go by and the FBI (his immune system) has now declared war on H. Pylori, making it prime enemy number one. This intensifies the inflammatory response in an attempt to kill the bad guy that increases the fluid build-up under the single-cell layer of tissue lining the arteries. This bulges the cell lining further into the lumen slightly blocking the flow of blood through the vessels. It also increases the smooth muscle tone and despite the doctor's increase in dosage over the past few years, John's blood pressure required another medication.

The vessel walls in the brain have been breached and the astrocytes are failing, allowing not only H. pylori to interact with microglial immune responses in the brain but have allowed other chemicals circulating in John's blood to enter the CNS – things that never should have passed. These new sources of inflammation in the brain have affected neural pathways and John now attributes his slight, worsening memory loss to his age.

Continue the story a few more years and see John lying in a hospital bed after placement of a stent or bypass surgery where the cardiologist found 90% blockage in several arteries. Picture John with early Dementia, peripheral neuropathy, anxiety, a growing depression, or MS. "We've done everything we could," may be a commonly heard phrase from his doctor at this point. But is that true?

Dr. Sherlock Holmes

Let's ask a couple questions:

1. Was CAUSE ever addressed?
2. Everything I've taught you to this point is NOT alternative; it's all in the literature. Why didn't anyone dig any deeper?
3. If CAUSE is just going to be ignored, is John EVER going to really get better?

Let's just pretend that John came into the office of competent physician, Dr. Sherlock Holmes before deciding to fill his prescriptions:

John enters with some legitimate concerns with his heart, loss of breath, sleep issues, memory loss, unclear thinking, and dizziness that the good doctor will need to address. After explaining the need to find the cause, John agrees to a thorough examination and series of functional labs which may include: Oxidized LDL (oxLDL), Homocysteine, high sensitivity C-Reactive Protein (hsCRP) which may indicate acute inflammation. Tests that may reveal oxidative stress include: 8-hydroxyguanosine (8-OHG) & 8-hydroxy-2'-deoxyguanosine (8-OHdG) – products of oxidized DNA and RNA; Malondialdehyde (MDA) – byproduct of lipid peroxidation; and Glutathione Superoxide Dismutase (SOD) – if decreased suspect oxidative stress.

As far as measuring blood lipid levels, the doctor, suspecting brain inflammation, wants to get more specific than just cholesterol, LDL and HDL levels: LDLs: Lipoprotein (a) is a 'regular' LDL with a protein structure attached. This combination increases the risk of CVD and endothelial damage. Levels are largely genetic but should be <30 mg/dL. Apolipoprotein B is a carrier protein that helps LDL deposit fat in arterial walls – levels should be <60 mg/dL. IDL (intermediate density lipoprotein) are VLDLs that are depositing some of their cholesterol and fat in the arteries. As VLDLs shed their fat, they become more dense and graduate to become an LDL. LDL-real (LDL-R) – all remaining LDLs. Some are small, some large. The smaller ones are more 'dangerous' even though they carry less cholesterol because they can better infiltrate damaged endothelium. In general: the smallest size LDL (LDL-B) is the most dangerous. LDL-A is least dangerous. VLDL or Triglycerides should be <75 mg/dL.

HDLs: HDL-2 – larger and more protective (especially HDL-2b); HDL-3 – smaller, less protective; Normally HDL is anti-oxidant and generally protective BUT…in the presence of a large amount of inflammation (like a chronic Autoimmune disorder), HDL can become oxidized that renders it useless.

An example of a more complete blood work-up for John then might include: Total Cholesterol, HDL Cholesterol and its sub factors, LDL Cholesterol and its sub factors, Triglycerides, Lipoprotein (a), Lipoprotein Ratios: LDL/HDL & Total/HDL, Ferritin, Fibrinogen, c-Reactive Protein (HS), Insulin ; Testosterone; Sex Hormone Binding

Globulin; Free Androgen Index; Magnesium, Homocysteine ; Coenzyme Q10; Lipid Peroxides. There's more but that suffices.

Tests to identify autoimmune dysfunction include: specific cytokine tests to measure increases in IL-1, IL-2, IL-6, IL-10; Heavy Metal toxicity testing; specific food antigen testing; environmental toxicity testing, and so on. I use Kinesiology testing and have kits for every known bio-toxin (virus, mold, fungus, parasite, bacteria) known to man so in our office we can find EXACTLY the cause of both endothelial and brain inflammation!

Whew, this is really getting boring with all these big words so let me summarize:

1. Never take medication based on lab work or symptoms that doesn't identify CAUSE. Using medication to manipulate lab values simply give the illusion of health. Don't go to Dr. David Copperfield, it's all a ruse.

2. There are many more specific labs, exams, and testing (including Kinesiology) that can be done that will EXACTLY point to one of the three causes of endothelial dysfunction/blood-brain barrier disruption. Find a Dr. Sherlock Holmes in your area!

3. You NEED to identify if you have a local inflammatory process, an oxidative stress response, or an autoimmune disorder that is causing the BBB disruption and the brain inflammation that follows in order to treat it properly. Medication will never cure you and identification of the possible antigen allows you to remove it and take steps to decrease inflammation and heal the brain.

Protective Measures that Heal the Blood-Brain Barrier

The following is a list of several OTHER things that everyone can do to protect against BBB disruption and heal the damage that already occurred. By "other" I mean that I am assuming that you are already correcting the CAUSE of endothelial damage that caused the astrocyte destruction.

1. Increase Endothelial Progenitor Cells (EPCs) – EPCs are similar to stem cells to your arteries. They rebuild and repair your tissue and need to be in high levels for regular, daily damage to be taken care of. Measuring them (lab test) is perhaps the greatest indicator of early impairment – low values equaling a greater risk. They are created in the cord blood and bone marrow similar to stem cells and are released and mobilized when vascular damage occurs. Think of EPCs as little carriers of MnSOD and Glutathione – two mighty anti-inflammatory chemicals that stimulate healing.

How do we increase EPCs?

a. EPCs increase with Growth Hormone (GH) release. All of us, even adults, release IGF-1, a precursor to GH while we sleep. Its purpose is to stimulate a Th1 (immune response) in the gut to kill off accumulated toxins in the intestinal tract from a hard day's work (especially necessary for those with poor HCl) and do other things associated with tissue repair like increase EPCs. The BEST way to stimulate IGF-1 production is to get a good night's sleep! NEVER take GH or GH stimulating hormones as they can stimulate cancer growth.

b. There are nutritional protocols that increase EPCs which include Resveratrol, Green Tea Extract (EGCGs), and products that increase Nitric Oxide: Omega-3 fatty acids, Garlic, ALA, NAC, Hawthorne, Pomegranate, gamma and delta Tocopherols, Tocotrienols, Vitamin C, Vitamin D, Vitamin K2-MK7, the B Vitamins, Flavonoids, CoQ-10, L-Arginine, Citrulline, Carnitine, Taurine, Celery, Pycnogenol, Grape Seed Extract, Hesperidin, Melatonin, NADH, Selenium, Bilberry, Turmeric, Quercetin, cruciferous vegetables, and Medicinal Mushrooms – just to name a few.

c. Perhaps the greatest way to increase EPCs is through exercise. The best choice of exercise is NOT sustained distance as in running five miles. To increase EPC production and protect yourself from BBB disruption, interval training is what you want to do – repetitions of 100% effort for a relatively short period of time followed by a repetition of 50% effort.

d. Of course, you MUST eliminate the things that decrease EPCs which includes the removing the source of inflammation and addressing the three responses I've covered – oxidative stress, inflammation, and autoimmune disorders.

2. Improve your diet to balance blood sugar swings, diabetic precursors, food sensitivities and toxic insults:

a. The best indicators of a pre-diabetic state include:

i. HbA1C – measures the percent of circulating hemoglobin (the cells responsible for delivering oxygen to the tissues) that are glycated, or 'stuck to glucose'. They are like sticky buns floating through your bloodstream! I like to see my patients at around 5.0 on their HbA1C.

ii. Oxidized LDL – as I discussed earlier, LDLs measured as a whole tell little of the type of LDL in circulation. We want to get more specific. Though there are several things that can oxidize both LDLs and HDLs, diabetes and pre-diabetes is one factor under your complete control.

iii. Another modification of LDLs is glycated LDLs. If glycated hemoglobin could be likened to circulating sticky buns, glycated LDLs could be circulating 'sticky lard'. I'm trying to give you a word picture that makes you a bit queasy. These glycated molecules attach to receptor sites on the endothelial wall called Pattern Recognition Receptors (PRRs) that then make your life miserable.

b. See my diet "Eating God's Way for your BBB" below:

NEW Eating God's Way for Your BBB

Meat (grass-fed organic ONLY – high in protein and Omega 3)

- NO meat for first _____ months
- meat bone soup or stock, liver and heart (must be organic)
- lamb, buffalo, elk, venison, beef, goat, veal
- jerky (organic with no chemicals, nitrates, or nitrites)
- beef or buffalo sausage (with no chemicals and preferably no pork casing)
- beef or buffalo hot dogs (with no chemicals and preferably no pork casing)

Fish (wild- caught ONLY, and the fish must be fish with fins and scales. Eg: No catfish)

- NO fish for first _____ months
- fish soup or stock, salmon, halibut, tuna, cod, scrod, grouper, haddock, walleye, panfish, lake fish
- trout, orange roughy, sea bass, snapper, sardines (canned in water or olive oil only), herring, sole, whitefish

Poultry (pastured, free-range and organic)

- NO poultry for first _____ months
- poultry bone soup or stock, chicken, Cornish game hen, guinea fowl, turkey, duck
- chicken or turkey bacon or sausage

Lunch Meat (organic, free range, and hormone free ONLY)

- NONE

Eggs (high omega-3/DHA or organic is best)

- chicken eggs (whole with yolk) UNLESS Egg intolerant

Dairy (organic and UN-Pasteurized (RAW) ONLY – NON if Dairy Intolerant!!!!)

- NO dairy for first _____ months
- Really NO Dairy for everyone is BEST unless RAW but that's hard to find
- homemade kefir made from raw goat's milk or raw cow's milk

- raw goat's milk hard cheeses, raw cow's milk hard cheeses
- goat's milk plain whole yogurt, organic cow's milk yogurt or kefir
- raw cream, raw butter if possible (or organic)

Fats and Oils (organic is best, you MUST EAT A LOT OF GOOD FAT)

- Oil: coconut oil, extra virgin (best for cooking) olive oil,
- Spread: Ghee butter; RAW butter
- Avocado (eat one every day), coconut milk/cream (canned), oil,
- PARENT OILS – Coconut oil, flax oil, borage oil, seed oils

Vegetables (organic fresh or frozen is best)

- ALL veggies are good – especially lower carb, organic (broccoli, artichokes, asparagus, beets, cauliflower)
- STRICTLY LIMIT white potatoes and corn (corn is really a grain), eat sweet potatoes instead

Fruits (organic fresh or frozen is best)

- Stone fruits are BEST – fruits with a pit
- LIMIT dried fruits (no sugar or sulfites), raisins, figs, dates, prunes; NO FRUIT JUICES!!!

*Grains and Starchy Carbohydrates (organic is best, and whole grains and flours are best if soaked for six to twelve hours before cooking) ***Brain-Based Therapy patients MUST stay off Gluten!!!*

- **NO GRAINS is best!!!!!!!!!!! Yes, that's right, I said NO GRAINS!**
- **Gluten-FREE** oats, rice, millet
- Pamela's Mix brand flour for baking, waffles, pancakes; use Quinoa
- UDI bread is a good gluten free brand that makes bread and muffins but it is high carbs!

Sweeteners (NO Artificial and NO High Fructose Corn Syrup!!!)

- Unheated raw honey; honey; date sugar; stevia; pure maple syrup; **NO ARTIFICIAL SWEETNERS**!!!!!!

Beans and Legumes (best if soaked for twelve hours)

- miso, lentils, tempeh, natto, black beans, kidney beans, navy beans, white beans, pinto beans, red beans
- split peas, garbanzo beans, lima beans, broad beans, black-eyed peas

Nuts and Seeds (organic, raw, and/or soaked is best)

- RAW almonds, pumpkin seeds, hemp seeds, flaxseeds, sunflower seeds, almond butter, tahini,
- hemp or pumpkin seed butter, sunflower butter, walnuts, macadamia nuts, pecans, hazelnuts, Brazil nuts

Condiments, Spices, and Seasonings (organic is best – MUST BE GLUTEN FREE)

- salsa (fresh or canned), tomato sauce (no added sugar), guacamole (fresh), NO soy sauce (use Bragg's Aminos)
- apple cider vinegar, raw salad dressings and marinades, herbs and spices (no added stabilizers)
- Herbamare seasoning, Celtic Sea Salt, sea salt, mustard, ketchup (no High Fructose Corn Syrup), salad dressings (no canola oil)
- marinades (no canola oil), omega-3 mayonnaise, natural extracts such as vanilla or almond

Beverages

- Reverse osmosis purified water; unsweetened herbal teas, raw vegetable or fruit juices, lacto-fermented beverages (like Kombucha – unless Candida issues), coconut water

*Limit Carbohydrates to less than 50 grams/day or less   *Detox Diets I recommend may severely limit some of the above for a period of time   *Consider Coffee Enemas to flush out the intestinal tract and cleanse the body   *Add ONLY supplements that Dr. Conners has instructed – never buy things from store!*Study and meditate on Scripture daily, focus on what is good, holy and righteous; keep away from the negative, bad thoughts and disease-oriented thinking. Focus on the PROCESS not the outcome.*

Changing the way your brain thinks

Neuro-Plasticity

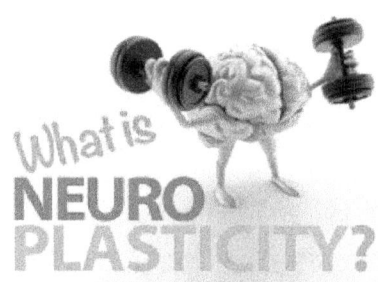

The brain has approximately 100 billion neurons with trillions of possible connections. It has been estimated that there are more synaptic connections in one human brain than there are stars in the known universe. This gives the brain virtually limitless processing power and a tremendous variability in this system. There are thousands of different neurotransmitters and the number of connections changes with activity. The type and the density of receptors can be regulated up or down. Hormones can influence the sensitivity of the cells and/or neurotransmitters and the number of synaptic connections can vary.

The human brain is extremely plastic, which means it is modifiable based on activity and experiences. It can change its shape, size, number of branches, and number of connections as well as the strength of its connections. Neurons in the brain are interconnected with many other neurons and, in turn, each neuron receives input from many synapses of its dendrites and cell body and, as stated earlier, communication through glial cells is now found to be possible.

The resulting neuronal loops contain neurons whose output signal may be either excitatory or inhibitory – they 'turn on' and 'turn off' impulses. Here's an example: Pain fibers in your body (let's use your feet as an example) are constantly firing from pressure receptors that travel pathways called 'small diameter afferents' (SDAs). These SDAs are constantly firing into the brain, without stopping. So how does the average (healthy) person NOT have constant pain? Well, there are other pathways that block this pain signal. One is the 'large diameter afferent' (LDA) pathway that gives collateral inhibitory signals to shut-down the pain signal. Another is called the 'descending inhibitory pain pathway' coming from the frontal lobe, firing to the spinal cord to where the SDAs enter a little way-station called Lamina 2. Here the descending inhibitory pathway squashes the pain signals so your feet don't hurt.

A fast tongue is a sign of a slow brain"
— Abu Fennek

TMI - Too much information? Stick with me here because I want you to think about this for a minute. If I have a problem with my LDAs and/or a problem with my descending inhibitory pain pathway, I *will* (not maybe) have chronic pain! But get this, it is NOT because I have a greater SOURCE of pain, it is because I cannot inhibit current 'normal' pain signals!

Okay, maybe I'm the only one that finds this fascinating but from a neurological point of view, these pathways can be tested. Moreover, they can (in most cases) be rehabbed!

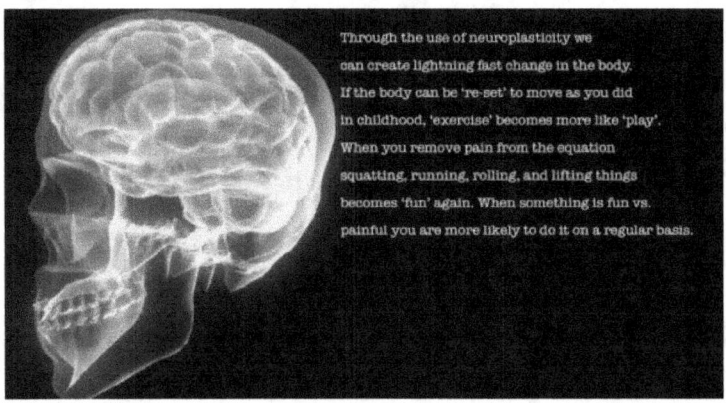

Through the use of neuroplasticity we can create lightning fast change in the body. If the body can be 're-set' to move as you did in childhood, 'exercise' becomes more like 'play'. When you remove pain from the equation squatting, running, rolling, and lifting things becomes 'fun' again. When something is fun vs. painful you are more likely to do it on a regular basis.

In Functional Neurology we say that if two neurons are excited together, they become linked functionally. In short, neurons that FIRE TOGETHER, WIRE TOGETHER. One can therefore make real, anatomical changes in neuronal pathways by purposefully firing nearby neuronal pools. Neurons stay alive through two necessary forces: Fuel and activation. If there is a decrease in either, the pathway dies!

Example: John has a decreased firing on his Dorso-lateral pre-frontal cortex (DLPFC) with symptoms of ADD/ADHD and many behavioral issues. We develop a program of stimulation of the DLPFC through Neurofeedback and a series of home brain-based therapies that will repeatedly fire into the DLPFC and "re-pave" the road. Of course, the cause must be corrected as well (source of inflammation, etc.).

When a neuron is stimulated, it will produce more protein for production of membrane, neurotransmitters, and organelles, like mitochondria. If you were to view the brains of people who frequently practice playing the violin under fMRI (functional MRI) they appear to have developed a larger area of their brain devoted to mapping their fingers. This change is directly related to the quantity and the quality of the practice they're performing – their brains are adapting in very real and necessary ways.

> "What the Net seems to be doing is chipping away my capacity for concentration and contemplation. Whether I'm online or not, my mind now expects to take in information the way the Net distributes it: in a swiftly moving stream of particles. Once I was a scuba diver in the sea of words. Now I zip along the surface like a guy on a Jet Ski."
> — Nicholas G. Carr, The Shallows: What the Internet is Doing to Our Brains

Author Mike Torres writes, "You can picture this yourself by imagining the flow of water through sand (I'm writing this from a beach in Kauai so excuse the metaphor – but I always find a mental motion picture is worth a thousand words!) When seawater first runs over the sand, there isn't a path for it to follow so it starts to form one for itself. As the water continues to flow over the sand, the pathway forms a real groove in the sand and gets deeper and more defined. It may start to branch off and take up more room in the sand if necessary, even reforming pathways on top of pathways that are no longer in use if it needs to. Once the pathways are formed, it becomes more difficult to change the water flow – and if the water ever stops flowing, the pathway will remain for some time in the hopes that it'll be used again at some point." (This is why picking something back up after some time of inactivity is easier than starting a new activity cold).

What we'll discuss in detail is that, in order to function and grow, brain cells need two things. One is fuel in the form of oxygen and glucose; and the second is stimulation (brain exercise). However, increasing fuel alone does not cause brain cells to grow; only stimulation does. As the brain cells grow in size, they require more fuel to have the ability to do more work.

If our brain cells have an abundance of fuel (oxygen and glucose), but we fail to stimulate it, the brain cells degenerate and die. Therefore, the most important element in growth of brain cells, and the growth of the brain itself, is based on increased stimulation. Although neurons have limitations in reproduction after birth, glial cells replicate based on increased metabolic demand of the neurons (increased stimulation). This increase in growth of glial cells allows the neurons to make more connections, which increases the ability and speed of the cell to transmit signal making both more efficient.

For decades, conventional science has held the position that 'the mind' is merely an illusion, a side-effect of electrochemical activity in the physical brain. Dr. Jeffrey Schwartz and Sharon Begley's work, "The Mind and the Brain", argues exactly the opposite: that the mind has a life of its own. Dr. Schwartz, a leading researcher in brain dysfunctions, and Wall Street Journal science columnist Sharon Begley demonstrate that the human mind is, "an independent entity that can shape and control the functioning of the physical brain." This helps us in the understanding of adult neuroplasticity–the brain's ability to be rewired not just in childhood, but throughout life.

Although the brain does provide itself with certain intense stimuli (e.g. dreams), when it comes to functioning in the real world, the brain is a stimulus-based system. It is dependent on outside sources (through receptors) for stimulation. Light, sound, vibration, odor, taste, pressure, heat and cold, and gravity would be examples. These are known as sensory input.

One of these senses, proprioception is the ability to be aware of one's body's position in space, body movements in relation to gravity, and to be aware of body movement in relationship to oneself. This information is collected from the environment in specialized structures known as mechanoreceptors. They are called receptors because they receive information. Receptors are specific (for the most part) for different forms of environmental stimuli. The retina has light receptors, rods, and cones; our ears possess sound and motion receptors, and our joints and muscles possess receptors for movement and gravity.

The more densely populated an area is in receptors, the more information or stimulation can be collected from that area. This density of receptors is not equally distributed throughout the body and has been represented in the silly picture below called the homunculus.

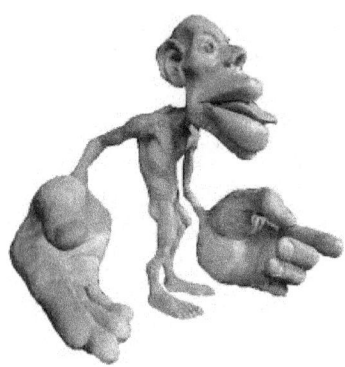

What has the lips of Mick Jagger, the body of Elijah Wood, the tongue of that guy from Kiss, and the hands of Michael Jordan? It's the homunculus. Although he looks like he should be either an exaggerated caricature of the president or someone out of Bill Cosby's imagination, the homunculus is a representation of the relationship between human body parts and the area of the brain responsible for them.

The homunculus comes in two varieties - sensory and motor. The sensory homunculus shows how much brain power is dedicated to sensing different body parts. It looks weird because the relative proportions of the body parts are not about physical size, but the number of related neural connections in the brain. The motor homunculus depicts the size of body parts based on the complexity of movements they can perform. When you think about how complex our hand and facial movements are, you can see why they're so big on the homunculus.

This is important as we develop specific brain-based therapies to purposefully and specifically stimulate neuronal centers. Firing receptors, fires the brain; given there are no lesions along the pathway, receptor stimulation is essential. Receptor stimulation is how our brain is mapped from day one! Babies that receive no physical stimulate (touch, love) fail to thrive not just because they emotionally fail but because of brain neuron death. "Tummy time", setting your baby on a blanket on the floor has a distinct purpose to stimulate brain function. I tell new parents to use their baby's feet and hands as 'worry stones', rubbing them constantly. You will have smarter and more well-balanced children should you purposefully stimulate skin receptors.

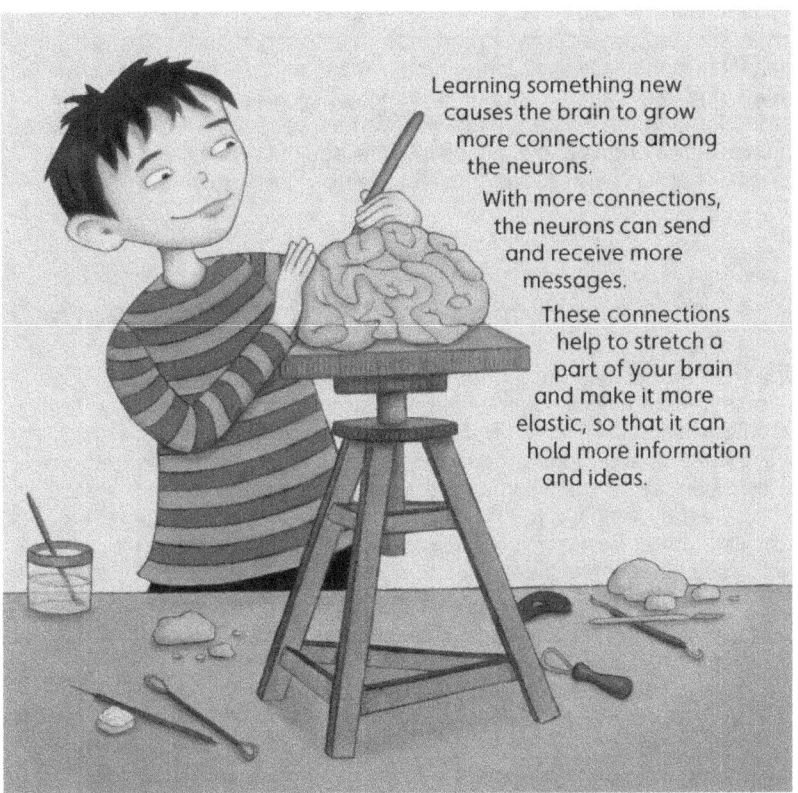

Learning something new causes the brain to grow more connections among the neurons.

With more connections, the neurons can send and receive more messages.

These connections help to stretch a part of your brain and make it more elastic, so that it can hold more information and ideas.

However, most environmental stimuli are not constant, not always available to stimulate the brain in the same way. Light, sound, taste, and temperature are all of variable frequency, duration, and intensity. For example, sunlight is only present during the day. The only constant source of stimulation from the environment is gravity. There is a purpose for this. We said that neurons need both stimuli and fuel and should there be just constant stimuli, fuel sources may run dry. Receptors also need a break.

Because gravity steadily exerts force on us whether we are standing, sitting, or lying down, and because we are perpetually forced to resist it by using muscles and joints, the amount of time it stimulates our brain based on frequency and duration is much greater than that of any other stimulus. Every movement we make stimulates the brain. Simply standing upright involves responses that not only allow us to see further, but also requires us to constantly resist gravity, even when we are standing still. This simple condition steadfastly increases stimulation to our brain therefore, accelerating its growth.

There are numerous studies on astronauts in zero gravity conditions that explain the absence of this constant stimulus as 'space madness'. Without constant stimulation the brain turns to mush. Neuroplasticity is so interesting; gravity and the effect it has on your muscle spindles and joints also accounts for healing tissue and bone growth. If a person fractures their leg and (as was the usual practice for decades) they are told to be as immobile as possible, they don't allow muscles to fire against gravity and healing is prolonged. Lessons: Get up and move; and don't let your children grow up to be astronauts.

Are Brain Problems Getting Worse?

Research has reported that the incidence of autism spectrum disorders and neurobehavioral developmental disabilities have been steadily on the rise. It also has been reported that today's children, in general, seem to have shorter attention span, decreasing scores in reading and language skills, and more impulsive behavior than they had as recently as ten years ago. Some studies show that these problems are becoming epidemic. Are they simply a result of poorer parenting skills, a greater number of dual income families, more unsupervised children, and a degenerative home environment or are these pieces that may play into a larger problem?

> *"And since nothing whatever happens to us outside our own brain; since nothing hurt us or gives us pleasure except within the brain, the supreme importance of being able to control what goes on in that mysterious brain is patent."*
> — *Arnold Bennett, How to Live on 24 Hours a Day*

Researchers have also been noting, both clinically and as reported in the literature, an increasing number of adults being diagnosed with Frontal Lobe disorders pointing, at least in part, that factor greater than sociological influences may be present.

Frontal Lobe disorders including Anxiety, Depression, ADD, ADHD and autism itself as well as other learning disabilities are growing at a staggering rate in the United States. In January of 2001, Newsday reported that 1 in 10 U.S. children have some sort of mental health problem, but less than 1 in 5 of them are being treated. This claim was made by the then Surgeon General of the United States, David Satcher, and reported in the same article.

A recent Wed MD article by Kathleen Doheny writes, "The number of children diagnosed with autism or related disorders has grown at what many call an alarming rate. In the 1970s and 1980s, about one out of every 2,000 children had autism. Today, the CDC estimates that one in 150 8-year-olds in the U.S. has an autism spectrum disorder, or ASD."

An article in March, 2013 USA Today stated, "Rates of all forms of autism in the U.S. may be substantially higher than previously estimated, according to a new government report that found that 1 out of every 50 school-age children – roughly one on every school bus – has the condition. That's dramatically higher than the 1 in 88 announced by a different government agency last year."

Alzheimer's disease has become the sixth leading cause of death in the United States. In 2013, Alzheimer's will cost the nation $203 billion. This number is expected to rise to $1.2 trillion by 2050. 1 in 3 seniors dies with Alzheimer's or another dementia.

Lyme disease, another neurological disorder, is the most commonly reported vectorborne illness in the United States – in 2012, it was the 7th most common Nationally Notifiable disease. Chronic Lyme disease (CLD) is a common, usually undiagnosed, cause of neurological dysfunction. According to current statistics, about 300,000 new cases of Lyme disease are diagnosed in the US each year—about 10 times higher than officially reported. While many still attribute Lyme transmission exclusively to ticks, the bacteria may also be spread by other insects, including mosquitoes, spiders, fleas, and mites. Diseases, such as Parkinson's, multiple sclerosis, cardiomyopathy, gastritis, and chronic fatigue, are all turning out to be expressions of chronic infections like CLD.

NBC News recently reported that, "for 40 million Americans, anxiety disorders are debilitating and omnipresent, and women are *twice* as likely to suffer as men." A 2010 article in Psychology Today reported that, "Rates of depression and anxiety among young people in America have been increasing steadily for the past fifty to seventy years. Today five to eight times as many high school and college students meet the criteria for diagnosis of major depression and/or an anxiety disorder as was true half a century or more ago." They went on to say that, "One thing we know about anxiety and depression is that they correlate significantly with people's sense of control or lack of control over their own lives." This is a Dorso-lateral prefrontal cortex function, i.e. it is a problem of the frontal lobe's connection to the deeper brain centers!

Numerous conditions that are reportedly left untreated include depression, considered one of the most common, attention deficit hyperactive disorder, and obsessive-compulsive disorder. Satcher stated, "Short of those diagnosable problems are problems that children have in their development and functioning very early." He suggested an overhaul of how mental health in children should be handled from training teachers and doctors, to better recognizing and understand these disorders, to doing more research and translating that research into effective treatment programs. Satcher is also quoted, "In any given year it is estimated that less than 1 in 5 of the children suffering from mental illness receive needed treatment."

> *Silencing the brain's ramblings gives the chance for wonderful thoughts to bloom."*
> — *Steven Redhead, The Solution*

Unfortunately, current 'treatment' typically consists of mind-altering medications. Those unfortunate enough to be in Satcher's 'treated' group are often left in a worse predicament than those left untreated. **We must address the cause**. We must overhaul our very definitions of care. While mood and mind-altering medications may be necessary for the temporary cessation of acute symptomology, they are not even addressing the reason for the brain imbalance and may even create a greater imbalance.

We can no longer ignore the problem. U.S. News and World Report recently stated that one in every six children in America suffers from problems such as autism, aggression, dyslexia, and attention deficit hyperactive disorder. New York, the number of children purportedly with learning disabilities jumped 55 percent from 132,000 to 204,000 between 1983 and 1996. California, reported cases of autism rose 210 percent from 3,864 to 100,995 between 1987 and 1998. "In the past decade, there has been a significant surge in the number of children diagnosed with autism throughout California," states the article. Even those who argue that it is the diagnosis of ASD's that has risen due to a heightened awareness don't dispute that the problem is indeed growing.

"The Centers for Disease Control and Prevention (CDC) estimates that about 1 in 88 children have been identified with an autism spectrum disorder (ASD). This data comes from the Autism and Developmental Disabilities Monitoring (ADDM) Network, which estimated the number of 8-year-old children with ASDs living in 14 communities throughout the United States in 2008. This new estimate marks a 23% increase since our last report in 2009, and a 78% increase since our first report in 2007." (Taken directly from the CDC website)

"Researchers say severe mental illness is more common among college students than it was a decade ago, with most young people seeking treatment for depression and anxiety. A study presented at the American Psychological Association found that the number of students on psychiatric medicines increased more than 10 percentage points over the last 10 years." (Depression On The Rise In College Students by Patti Neighmond, January 17, 2011)

Peter Gray in an article entitled, "Freedom to Learn - The roles of play and curiosity as foundations for learning," states, "Rates of depression and anxiety among young people in America have been increasing steadily for the past fifty to seventy years. Today five to eight times as many high school and college students meet the criteria for diagnosis of major depression and/or an anxiety disorder as was true half a century or more ago. This increased psychopathology is not the result of changed diagnostic criteria; it holds even when the measures and criteria are constant.

The most recent evidence for the sharp generational rise in young people's depression, anxiety, and other mental disorders comes from a just-released study headed by Jean Twenge at San Diego State University. Twenge and her colleagues took advantage of the fact that the *MMPI*--the Minnesota Multiphasic Personality Inventory, a questionnaire used to assess a variety of mental disorders--has been given to large samples of college students throughout the United States going as far back as 1938, and the *MMPI-A* (the version used with younger adolescents) has been given to samples of high school students going as far back as 1951."

These results are consistent with other studies, using a variety of indices, which also point to dramatic increases in anxiety and depression--in children as well as in adolescents and young adults--over the last five or more decades. Unfortunately, most individuals with such disorders and the health care professionals treating them do not have a good understanding of the etiology of the dysfunction. They do not understand what is wrong with their brain and often blame themselves, genetics, society, or think of themselves as "bad" people.

Chapter Three

So what's Wrong?

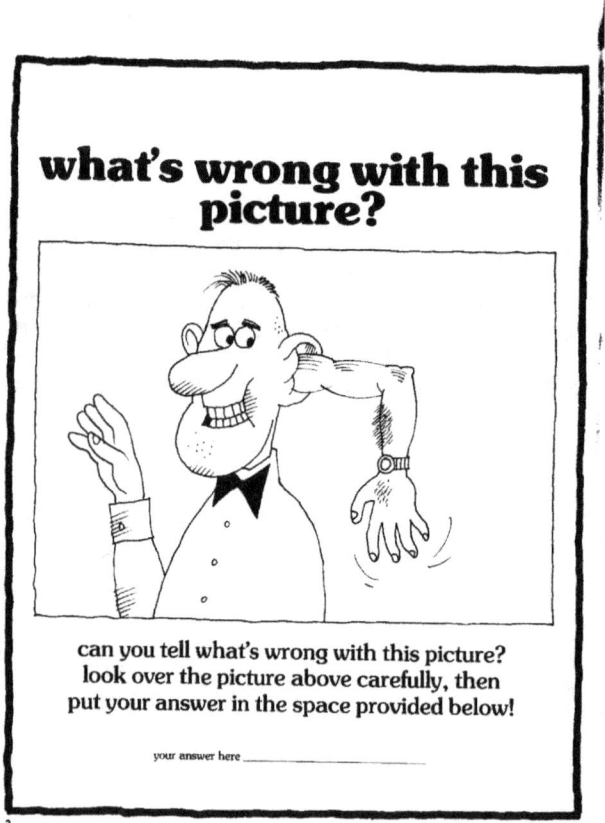

Things aren't always so obvious! But the problem doesn't go away by pretending that it doesn't exist. Drugs may numb the symptoms but they rarely correct the cause.

What are the 'causes'? Is there one secret supplement of which we are deficient? Is it all to be blamed on vaccinations, medications, parents, schools? There are no easy answers but, most assuredly, there are a multitude of factors that play into the problem.

Functional Delays

It doesn't take a social scientist to observe that children spend less time out on their bikes or roller skates, climbing trees or playing ball then a generation ago. They are inside watching TV, playing video or computer games, on Facebook and substituting 'false social networking' for the real thing. Adults fall into the same trap. A generation ago, people were intimately connected to a church, a club, and generally more social at work. The computer revolution has isolated us, segregated us, and turned us into left-brain stimulation junkies.

Parents don't talk to, read to, or spend time with their children as much as they did ten years ago. The stresses of modern day 'keep up with the Jones' mentality and the seeming obsession Americans have with new cars and the latest toys has changed so dramatically over the past two generations that it is an oddity for a family to be without a cell phone, iPod, Wii, or the like. The baby-sitter for both our children and our own deficiency in socialization is often the television, video games or the computer. Right-brain, imaginative play and creative communication falls by the wayside.

> *I never came upon any of my discoveries through the process of rational thinking.*
> *-Albert Einstein*

Jane Healy in her book "Endangered Minds, Why Children Don't Think and What We Can Do About It", quotes many interviews with teachers and some interesting studies with startling statistics. As an educator and administrator with 30 years experience, she comments that modern children seem to have "changing brains." Healey suggests that our current crisis in education and the growing problem with behavior has deep roots. Healy argues that contemporary society systematically under-nourishes the growing brains of our children at key developmental junctures. The predominance of two income families leads to a pattern of haphazard child care and a diminishing the number of opportunities for children to learn basic conversation skills. Television and video games absorb the time of children to the exclusion of reading and other forms of play, preempting important exercises in imagination and interactive communication. Even the much revered "Sesame Street" encourages a short attention span and fails to address the real educational needs of preschoolers. Likewise, trendy educational experiments designed to accelerate learning are often 'out of phase' with the needs of young brains. She argues that poverty exacerbates these problems for a growing number of children. As a result, our society fails to foster the physical development of young brains necessary for sophisticated command of language, analytic rigor, and sustained thought. In addition to her attack on "Sesame Street," Healy offers a clear challenge to true believers in phonics, cultural literacy, and other popular panaceas. She also expands the scope of analysis beyond the boundaries of the schoolyard, recognizing that the process of education involves broader social and life-style questions.

Healey writes, "Children were likable, fun to be with, intuitive, and often amazingly self aware." Today, in her estimation, they seem harder to teach, less tuned to verbal material both spoken and written. She discovered, "many admitted they didn't read very much, sometimes even the required homework." They struggle with or avoid writing assignments while teachers anguish over the results. One of the teachers she interviewed stated, "I feel like children have one foot out the door with whatever they are doing, they are incredibly easily distracted. I think there may have been a shift in the last five years."

Teachers interviewed by Healy felt that children today come to class with fewer social skills, less language ability, less ability to listen, and less motor ability and that in general, a frightening majority of children's attention spans have degenerated over recent years. Objective support for these reported conclusions is supported in the literature by numerous studies. One may conclude that sedentary lifestyles, increased television/computer viewing, and busy parents at least are partial causes of these dramatic statistical changes in cognitive, motor, and academic performance of present day western school aged children.

Developmental Profile

The Institutes for the Achievement of Human Potential has created a *Developmental Profile* as a delineation of the significant stages of child brain development through which children pass as they progress from birth to six years. The purpose of *The Developmental Profile* is to reduce the thousands of accomplishments that a child enjoys to those functions that are actually *causes* rather than mere results of other functions. It is a clear and reliable tool for measuring the degree of ability or disability—and rate of progress—of brain-injured and well children.

In the past, it was believed that this progression was predestined and unalterable as a result of genetic inheritance superimposed upon a rigid schedule of time and sequence.

Brain Stage	Time Frame	Visual Competence	Auditory Competence	Tactile Competence
VII Sophisticated Cortex	Superior 36 mon. Average 72 mon. Slow 144 mon.	Reading with total understanding	Understanding of complete vocabulary & proper sentences	Tactile Identification of objects
VI Primitive Cortex	Superior 18 mon. Average 36 mon. Slow 72 mon.	Identification of visual symbols and letters within experience	Understanding of 2000 words and simple sentences	Ability to determine characteristics of objects by tactile means
V Early Cortex	Superior 9 mon. Average 18 mon. Slow	Differentiation of similar but unlike simple visual symbols	Understanding of 10 to 25 words and two couplets	Tactile differentiation of similar but unlike objects

Brain Stage	Time Frame			
	36 mon.			
IV Initial Cortex	Superior 6 mon. Average 12 mon. Slow 24 mon.	Convergence of vision resulting in simple depth perception	Understanding of two words of speech	Tactile understanding of the third dimension in objects which appear to be flat
III Midbrain and Subcortical Areas	Superior 3.5 mon. Average 7 mon. Slow 14 mon.	Appreciation of detail within a configuration	Appreciation of meaningful sounds	Appreciation of gnostic sensation
II Brain Stem and Early Subcortical Areas	Superior 1 mon. Average 2.5 mon. Slow 5 mon.	Outline perception	Vital response to threatening sounds	Perception of vital sensation
I Early Brain Stem and Cord	Superior Birth to .5 mon. Average Birth to 1 mon. Slow Birth to 2 mon.	Light reflex	Startle reflex	Babinski reflex

The work of the staff of *The Institutes* from 1940 to the present has shown that this is untrue and that the order in which the significant stages take place is a function of brain development, as successively higher brain stages are brought into play. The time schedule is highly variable and depends, not upon genetic factors, but rather upon the frequency, intensity and duration of the stimuli provided to the brain by the child's environment, which is notably and most often his family.

The purpose and goal of taking both children and adults that have brain-based signs and symptoms through the steps of development are to re-train that brain, taking advantage of neuroplasticity. You are literally re-training or re-mapping neural pathways. This is the essence of Brain-Based Therapies.

Brain Stage	Time Frame	Mobility Competence	Language Competence	Manual Competence
VII Sophisticated Cortex	Superior 36 mon. Average 72 mon. Slow 144 mon.	Using a leg in a skilled role which is consistent with the dominant hemisphere	Complete vocabulary and proper sentence structure	Using a hand to write which is consistent with the dominant hemisphere
VI Primitive Cortex	Superior 18 mon. Average 36 mon. Slow 72 mon.	Walking and running in complete cross pattern	2000 words of language and short sentences	Bimanual function with one hand in a skilled role
V Early Cortex	Superior 9 mon. Average 18 mon. Slow 36 mon.	Walking with arms freed from the primary balance role	10 to 25 words of language and two couplets	Cortical opposition bilaterally and simultaneously
IV Initial Cortex	Superior 6 mon. Average 12 mon. Slow 24 mon.	Walking with arms used in a primary balance role most frequently at or above shoulder height	Two words of speech used spontaneously and meaningfully	Cortical opposition in either hand
III Midbrain and Subcortical Areas	Superior 3.5 mon. Average 7 mon. Slow 14 mon.	Creeping on hands and knees, culminating in cross pattern creeping	Creation of meaningful sounds	Prehensile grasp
II Brain Stem and Early Subcortical	Superior 1 mon. Average 2.5 mon. Slow	Crawling in the prone position culminating in cross pattern crawling	Vital crying in response to threats of life	Vital release

Areas	5 mon.			
I Early Brain Stem and Cord	Superior Birth to .5 mon. Average Birth to 1 mon. Slow Birth to 2 mon.	Movement of arms and legs without bodily movement	Birth cry and crying	Grasp reflex

The above table represents the stages of both sensory and motor development, as described in *The Institutes Developmental Profile* which was developed by the Institutes and all credit belongs to them.

When you look over the above charts, you will see that the two charts together are divided into six columns (three columns per chart).

They are:

1. **Mobility** competence (*gross motor movement*)
2. **Language** competence (*speech*)
3. **Manual** competence (*use of the hands*)
4. **Visual** competence (*seeing*)
5. **Auditory** competence (*hearing*)
6. **Tactile** competence (*feeling*)

The first three functions are *motor* functions found on the second chart; the last three are *sensory* functions from the first chart. The motor cortex is found primarily in the frontal lobe and the sensory is primarily parietal lobe. Both left and right frontal and parietal lobes function in balance to produce a normal developmental progression.

We begin to understand that, in the course of development, should a child experience any source of inflammation in a neural area, developmental progression may cease.

For each of the columns above, there are seven different colored rows. The bottom row, red, represents the child's brain function at birth. For example, in the manual column is the *grasp reflex*. In the visual column is the *light reflex*. In the auditory column is the *startle reflex*. The next row, orange, represents the next stage of brain development (*achieved in the average child by the age of 2.5 months*). For example, in the visual column we will find the ability to see outlines. In the language column, we will find the ability to cry more seriously in response to things that the baby finds threatening. The rows keep going, to yellow (*seven months*), green (*twelve months*), blue (*eighteen months*), indigo (*three years*), and lastly violet (*six years*). (credit given to The Institutes, see their website for more information and to order materials)

Though these charts may be listed as milestones, every child is unique and ONLY competent neurological and metabolic testing adequately determines problems and causes.

The most important thing to remember is this: IT ALL CAN BE CORRECTED!

The Metabolic Connection

Based on reports from caregivers, case studies, and observation of patients with schizophrenia and children with severe behavioral disorders, Dohan hypothesized (Dohan et al., 1969; 1984; Dohan, 1966a; 1966b; 1969; 1970; 1979; 1980a; 1980b; 1988) that **gluten and dairy foods might worsen these behaviors**. He noted that in many cases, a restricted diet could lead to significant improvement or recovery from these disorders.

Dr. Maios Hadjivassiliou of the United Kingdom, a recognized world authority on gluten sensitivity, has reported in the journal, The Lancet, that "gluten sensitivity can be primarily and at times, exclusively a neurological disease." That is, people can manifest gluten sensitivity by having issues with brain function without any gastrointestinal problems whatsoever. Dr. Hadjivassiliou indicates that the antibodies that a person has when they are gluten sensitive can be directly and uniquely toxic to the brain through what has become known neurologically as the gluteo-morphine receptors. These are found in the gut and fire directly to the same areas that morphine do. Therefore people with gluten sensitivities are affected primarily in the brain, not the gut.

The mind is its own place, and in itself
Can make a heaven of hell, a hell of heaven.
-John Milton (1608-1674), Paradise Lost

Since his original investigations in 1996, the recognition that gluten sensitivity can lead to disorders of brain function has led to a virtual explosion of scientific papers describing this relationship. A simple Google scholar search will reveal over 2000 peer-reviewed, scientifically based research articles on the effects of gluten and gluten peptides on the brain so tell your ignorant doctor who says it's a 'fad diet' to leave his golf clubs in the car and crack open a research journal and move into the 21st century.

Researchers in Israel have noted neurological problems in 51 percent of children with gluten sensitivity and further, describe a link between gluten sensitivity and attention deficit/hyperactivity disorder (ADHD). As authors in a recent issue of the journal, Pediatrics, stated in their research, "This study suggests that the variability of neurologic disorders that occur in celiac disease is broader than previously reported and includes softer and more common neurologic disorders including chronic headache, developmental delay, hypotonia and learning disorders or ADHD."

The link between gluten sensitivity and problems with brain function, including learning disabilities, difficulty staying on task and even memory dysfunction, is actually not that difficult to understand. Gluten sensitivity is caused by elevated levels of antibodies against a component of gluten, the protein gliadin. This antibody (anti-gliadin antibody) combines with gliadin when a person is exposed to any gluten containing food like wheat, barley, spelt, malt, or rye. Testing for the antibody can be performed in any doctor's office through either doing a stool test (through Enterolab) or a blood test for the gliadin peptides (through Cyrex Labs). When the antibody combines with this protein, specific genes are turned on in a special type of immune cell in the body.

When these genes are turned on, inflammatory chemicals are created called cytokines, which are directly detrimental to brain function. In fact, elevated cytokines are seen in such devastating conditions as Alzheimer's disease, Parkinson's disease, multiple sclerosis and even autism. Basically, the brain does not like inflammation and responds quite negatively to the presence of cytokines. Another problem with anti-gliadin antibody is that it can directly combine with specific proteins found in the brain. Specific brain proteins can look like the gliadin protein found in gluten-containing foods and the anti-gliadin antibody just can't tell the difference. This direct role of anti-gliadin antibody in combining with specific proteins in the brain has been described for decades and again leads to the formation of cytokines, the chemical mediators of inflammation. This is an example of turning on genes that ultimately function in a negative way in relation to brain health and function.

The 10 Most Common Symptoms of Gluten Sensitivity and Celiac Disease

- Brain fog
- Fatigue
- Headaches and/or migraines
- GI distress such as: abdominal pain and bloating, gas, queasiness, acid reflux, vomiting, constipation, and diarrhea
- Weight loss or weight gain
- Depression, irritability, listlessness, and emotional instability
- Joint pain, tingling, or numbness in the legs, arms, and hands
- Acne, eczema, and other skin rashes
- Hair loss
- Hashimoto's disease and other autoimmune disorders

Jane Anderson, in her 2012 article titled, Gluten-Related Neurological Symptoms and Conditions writes, "Neurological illnesses such as epilepsy, depression and anxiety also are common in those who react to gluten. In addition, a serious autoimmune condition called gluten ataxia affects a small number of people.

Finally, there are some hints that conditions such as schizophrenia and bipolar disorder also may be affected by gluten intake in a few individuals. However, it's not yet clear from the research who might be affected, and whether a gluten-free diet can help some people."

For several years, the biochemical explanation for this phenomenon remained unclear. However, several other studies seemed to bear out this observation until recently, using more advanced laboratory technology, researchers revealed abnormal peptides (portions of a gluten protein complex) in the urine of schizophrenics and autistics.

Peptides are pieces of proteins that are not completely broken down into individual amino acids. Think of entire gluten protein (gliadin) as a brick wall. What is supposed to happen to every protein consumed is that the 'brick wall' is broken into its individual bricks (amino acids) so they can cross the gut wall. This is what is known as digestion.

Reichelt has observed that these peptides, which are several amino acids long, have sequences that match those of opioid peptides (casomorphin and gliadomorphin). The known dietary sources of these **opiate peptides** are casein (from milk) and gliadin or gluten (from cereal grains). He has since conducted several studies examining this finding (Knivsberg et al., 2002; 2001; Pedersen et al., 1999; Reichelt et al., 1996; Seim & Reichelt, 1995), as have several other researchers (Garvey, 2002; Buckley, 1998), including Paul Shattock (Whiteley & Shattock, 2002) in England. The best evidence for this correlation lies in the many case reports of improvement or recovery of children with ASD on this diet.

The greatest discovery of my generation is that man can alter his life simply by altering his attitude of mind.
-William James (1842-1910)

For those following the science of the "gut microbiome," immune-brain and gut-brain relationships, it's easy to understand these relationships. Our immune system and our so-called "gut bugs" – the billions of microorganisms that live in our GI tract –have huge impacts on our health. "There are strong connections between the immune system and the brain, which are mediated through multiple physiological symptoms," senior author Laura Cousino Klein, associate professor of biobehavioral health and human development and family studies, said in a statement. "A majority of the pain receptors in the body are located in the gut, so by adhering to a gluten-free, casein-free (GF/DF) diet, you're reducing inflammation and discomfort that may alter brain processing, making the body more receptive to ASD therapies."

In a new Penn State survey of nearly 400 parents of ASD children on a GF/DF diet, it seemed to make a difference what choices parents made. Children who eliminated both gluten – the protein in wheat, rye, spelt, malt, and barley as well as the milk protein (casein) from their diet, and who stuck with it six months or more, seemed to do the best. Gluten is in more than wheat, and casein is in more than milk and cheese, so this takes hard work and discipline, but for many it seems to pay off. Some parents of children with autism as well as adults with autism themselves, report even greater benefit from eliminating fast-metabolizing starches, like sugars, grains and starchy vegetables including potatoes, which may feed noxious gut bugs.

According to a paper published in Natural News, "Approximately 10 percent of people with Celiac disease develop neurologic symptoms, according to the Center for Peripheral Neuropathy. Ataxia describes a neurologic condition characterized by jerky movements and an awkward gait. Gluten ataxia specifically describes a neurologic condition caused by a gluten sensitivity that leads to a wide range of symptoms, including:

- Difficultly concentrating
- Loss of balance
- Frequent falls
- Visual disturbances
- Trouble walking
- Tremors
- Trouble judging distances

In people with gluten sensitivity, eating foods with the gluten protein triggers an autoimmune reaction. The body attacks the gluten with antibodies in the same way that antibodies attack viruses. This damages the intestines. Intestinal damage inhibits absorption of nutrients, often leading to nutrient deficiencies.

Vitamin deficiencies could (also) be to blame for gluten ataxia, according to an article in the Feb/Mar 2011 issue of Living Without magazine. Another explanation is that something in the brain is similar enough to gluten that the antibodies released to attack gluten also attack the brain.

Neuropathy, or peripheral neuropathy, describes a range of disorders characterized by nerve damage to one or more nerves outside of the brain and spinal cord. Often the cause of the neuropathy is unknown, though autoimmune diseases and vitamin deficiencies are some of the potential causes, according to the Mayo Clinic. Gluten neuropathy is when the autoimmune response is the root cause of the nerve damage.

A study published in Muscle & Nerve journal in December 2006 found that participants with neuropathy who followed a gluten-free diet showed significant improvement in symptoms after one year. The control group reported worsening of symptoms. A few years ago I had a young female patient with idiopathic foot drop (loss of upward flexion of her foot) noticed by frequent tripping on the soccer field. After a complete examination process, I was surprised that gluten sensitivity was her only finding and elimination of all gluten and possible gluten-contaminated foods completely resolved her problems.

It is also thought that food peptides (partially digested pieces of proteins that never should have passed the gut wall) might be responsible for toxic effects at the level of the central nervous system by interacting with neurotransmitters. For more information on gluten sensitivities and celiac disease, I suggest you visit: www. theglutensyndrome.net and www.thedr.com.

The multi-headed monster of food sensitivities are all because of BRAIN INFLAMMATION. Nutritional therapies are varied. There are dietary changes, nutritional supplements, herbal medicines, and homeopathy that are the most commonly used and accepted forms of therapy for children and adults. It is important that proper testing be done to determine the individual's specific source of inflammation.

Food Allergies, Behavior and Gut Health

There has been extensive research examining the brain-intestinal connection. It is fairly well documented that the GALT (gut associated lymphoid tissue) is associated with an individual's absorption and immune responsiveness. It is also thought that in various individuals who damage these barrier cells can become overly sensitive to normally good foods, end up with specific nutritional deficiencies, and suffer from poor brain regulation. The gastrointestinal system, as a result, becomes less efficient at filtering allergens and larger molecules that may be associated with allergic responses pass through into the blood. This has been termed intestinal permeability or leaky gut.

The lining of the intestines is covered with villi that resemble shag carpeting. Its purpose is to give an increased surface area for nutrient absorption. The cells also act as a barrier that normally only allows properly digested fats, proteins, and starches to pass through and enter the bloodstream. It allows substances to pass in several ways.

I like nonsense; it wakes up the brain cells
-Dr. Seuss

Chloride, potassium, magnesium, sodium and free fatty acids diffuse through intestinal cell membranes. Amino acids, fatty acids, glucose, minerals, and vitamins also cross through cells, but they do it by another mechanism called active transport. There's a third way substances can pass through. The spaces in between the cells that line the intestinal villi are normally sealed connections. These tight junctions are called desmosomes. When the intestinal lining becomes damaged, the junctions loosen and allow unwanted larger molecules in the intestines to pass through.

The 'barrier' has been breached. These unwanted substances are seen by the immune system as foreign (because they aren't normally present in blood) and an enemy attack ensues. Here's what you need to know about the primary function of what's called the initial, TH1 response of the immune system – it KILLS things. Your immune system turns-on against foreign invaders to do one thing – kill them. This is your defense system that is to protect you from pathogens. Can you sense a problem here? Are peptides from gluten or casein living organisms (pathogens) that will be killed by an immune attack?

This becomes a major problem. In an immune reaction, the initial, killer cell response (a TH1 reaction) is to kill the pathogen. Should the victory not be achieved, the TH1 response suppresses and a TH2 response fire to trigger a production of antibodies against said pathogen. In leaky gut syndrome invasion of non-living substances (continue with our gluten example but other invaders can be equally a problem) fire a TH1 reaction that will never result in death of the antigen (we call anything that sparks a TH1 response an antigen in an immune reaction) because IT'S NOT ALIVE.

It makes sense to me – your immune system can be the epitome of health and it will never win if it's trying to kill something that can never die! Then, if your healthy immune system (TH2 response) makes antibodies to the peptides, you are in big trouble. Now you'll have a sustained immune attack against the peptides where it finds them.

When the intestinal lining becomes further damaged, even larger substances, such as disease-causing bacteria (like Helicobacter pylori), other undigested food particles, and toxins, pass directly through the damaged cells. Again, the immune system is alarmed and antibodies and substances called cytokines are released and the cycle continues!

Chemo Brain

As the American Cancer Society states, "For years cancer survivors have worried about, joked about, and been frustrated by the mental cloudiness they sometimes notice before, during, and after cancer treatment commonly called chemo brain. Patients have been aware of chemo brain for some time, but only recently have studies been done that could help to explain it.

Doctors have known for years that radiation treatment to the brain can cause thinking and memory problems. Recently, they have found that chemotherapy is linked to some of the same kinds of problems. Research shows that some cancer drugs can cause certain kinds of changes in the brain. But it also shows that chemo and radiation aren't the only things that can cause thinking and memory problems in people with cancer.

Though the brain usually recovers over time, the sometimes vague yet distressing mental changes cancer patients notice are real not imagined. They might last a short time, or they might go on for years. These changes can make people unable to go back to their school, work, or social activities, or make it so that it takes a lot of mental effort to do so. Chemo brain changes affect everyday life for many people, and more research is needed to help prevent and cope with them.

Here are just a few examples of what patients call chemo brain:

- Forgetting things that they usually have no trouble recalling (memory lapses)
- Trouble concentrating (they can't focus on what they're doing, have a short attention span, may "space out")
- Trouble remembering details like names, dates, and sometimes larger events
- Trouble multi-tasking, like answering the phone while cooking, without losing track of one task (they are less able to do more than one thing at a time)
- Taking longer to finish things (disorganized, slower thinking and processing)
- Trouble remembering common words (unable to find the right words to finish a sentence)

Doctors and researchers call chemo brain "mild cognitive impairment." Most define it as being unable to remember certain things and having trouble finishing tasks or learning new skills. But some doctors call it chemo brain only if it doesn't go away or get better

over time. How long it lasts is a major factor in how much it affects a person's life."
(www.cancer.org also see www.stopfightingcancer.com)

Chemotherapy is a poison, plain and simple. The protective barrier that is supposed to keep dangerous toxins and pathogens from entering the brain (the blood-brain barrier) is made up of astrocytes that are damaged by, wait for it....chemicals! Chemotherapy patients that have already damaged blood-brain barriers from previous toxic exposure (GMOs, pesticides, herbicides, additives, excitotoxins...) have a greater susceptibility to neurological effects from chemotherapy. Those entering chemotherapy with an intact brain barrier will, most assuredly, have damaged to the barrier from the chemo.

Neurofeedback Cures Chemo Brain

"Social psychologist Jean Alvarez, a breast cancer survivor, struggled with the condition for years. In 2007, the Lakewood resident turned to neurofeedback when nothing else seemed to help her get rid of the two symptoms she said were "left over" from

> *An idle brain is the devil's workshop.*
> *-Old English Proverb*

chemotherapy treatment that ended years earlier," reports Cleveland.com, as Sun News publication in an article titled, "Neurofeedback helps relieve chemo brain symptoms, Cleveland researcher finds".

I'll quote this interesting piece as it was inspirational to me and influential in our decision to invest in this equipment for our clinic. "Electroencephalogram, or EEG, biofeedback, otherwise known as neurofeedback, is a noninvasive treatment that provides information on and measures changes in a person's brain-wave activity. The brain "self-corrects" by using the feedback to reorganize.

Traditional neurofeedback pinpoints a specific area of the brain in need of correction. But no one knows what the electrical "signature" of chemo brain is, so Alvarez used another type of neurofeedback equipment that addresses the brain as an integrated system, making the specific location of the problem less important.

Resistant to the suggestion of her physician at the time to undergo neuropsychological testing, Alvarez instead decided to pursue neurofeedback after revisiting something she had previously read about the technique.

Not only did Alvarez find relief, but after 10 treatments, she felt as good as she had before she began chemotherapy. That led her to design a research study to see if her success could be replicated. She hoped to provide relief to others more quickly than if they waited for symptoms to dissipate on their own, months or years later.

The small study looked at the impact of neurofeedback on lessening post-cancer cognitive impairment, or PCCI. Her study was published online April 12 in the journal Integrative Cancer Therapies. The type of neurofeedback employed in the study was a brief interruption in music that the study subject was listening to. This newer approach to neurofeedback, Alvarez wrote, trains the whole brain by having participants "let go" instead of engaging actively or consciously with the instrument providing that feedback.

Alvarez, director of research at the newly incorporated Cleveland-based Applied Brain Research Foundation of Ohio, began enrolling breast cancer patients for the study in early 2010. Twenty-three women, who ranged in age from 43 to 70 and who had completed treatment for breast cancer, received biofeedback in 45-minute sessions, twice a week for 10 weeks. The time from the last chemotherapy treatment to the start of the biofeedback ranged from six months to five years.

The study participants were given four different self-reporting tests for 10 weeks that measured cognitive function; fatigue, energy level and quality of life; sleep quality and disturbances; and somatization (when mental factors such as stress cause physical symptoms), depression and anxiety. Over a second 10-week period, the participants received neurofeedback twice a week, for 33 minutes a session, and continued the self-reporting tests. Four weeks after the last neurofeedback session, the women completed one final self-reporting test.

What Alvarez found was that the treatment did help relieve symptoms of PCCI, or chemo brain, and it did help other patients return to the level of function they had prior to starting chemotherapy.

Chemo brain symptoms were reversed in 21 of the 23 women.

"I was hoping to see all of those good results, but I'm not sure I was expecting to see them," Alvarez said. "Almost everyone improved and returned to normal levels. That was surprising and gratifying."

Not all of the study participants showed benefits right away, or at the same rate, she said. Some started noticing a change after a half-dozen sessions, while a few didn't begin seeing improvement until toward the end of their participation, Alvarez said.

For some women, sleep quality improved first; in others, symptoms of depression lessened, she said, adding, "It's a pretty individual process."

A real difference for one patient

Diagnosed with breast cancer in late 2008, Dianne Borowski of Bay Village completed chemotherapy in July 2009. In February 2010 she contacted Alvarez and enrolled in the study soon afterward.

"I was having quite a bit of it [chemo brain]," said Borowski, 71, who was plagued by memory and sleep troubles. When she heard about the trial and that it was looking for volunteers, "I thought, 'My goodness. This is wonderful.' "

Relief from the sessions was not instantaneous, she said. But as time went by, she started to notice a real difference. She started misplacing things less frequently. Her sleep improved. She no longer had to search for words to express herself. "I was amazed at the process and how it started to work," she said. Borowski says her chemo brain flares up occasionally if she's under a lot of stress, but so far it hasn't returned to her pre-chemotherapy levels.

Researchers continue to shed light on the effect that chemo brain -- given that name only in the past dozen years or so -- has on cancer survivors.

Last week, the Journal of the National Cancer Institute published online a study from the University of California, Los Angeles. Researchers who evaluated 189 early-stage breast cancer patients post-treatment (radiation and/or chemotherapy) found a strong link between patients' self-reported complaints of changes in memory and thinking and data from neuropsychological testing that showed those changes.

You know you've got to exercise your brain just like your muscles.
-Will Rogers

A study that appeared in the Journal of Clinical Oncology in early 2012 found lingering cognitive effects of chemotherapy in some breast cancer patients as long as 20 years after treatment.

It is the heart and not the brain
That to the highest doth attain.
-Longfellow, The Building of the Ship

Over the summer at the annual American Society of Clinical Oncology meeting, Cleveland Clinic's Taussig Cancer Institute oncologist Dr. Halle Moore presented the results of a small pilot study that showed the EEG to be a good measuring tool in documenting the impact of chemo brain on changes in brain function.

"Chemo brain is real," said Dr. Fremonta Meyer, a psychiatrist at the Dana Farber Cancer Institute in Boston and co-author of Alvarez's study who helped interpret the data.

Among the patients she sees are those with post-cancer cognitive problems that may sound like the effects of normal aging or menopause. But difficulty finding words, short-term memory loss, problems sleeping and the inability to multitask effectively are all things that can be the result of chemo brain, she said.

One of the big shortcomings in the literature dealing with chemo brain has been the lack of solutions to the defined problem, Meyer said. "We now have another intervention that we can [potentially] offer to patients, which I think is huge," she said.

It wasn't just a placebo effect

While questions can be raised about whether the soothing qualities of the neurofeedback worked as a placebo and served to calm the participants or whether it was the neurofeedback that led to cognitive improvements, the researchers maintain that the results are hard to attribute to a placebo effect alone.

They point to several factors that underscore the validity and reliability of neurofeedback, among them:

> • Analysis that focused on improvement following the self-reporting tests, after a placebo effect would have been present.

> • Measuring the neurofeedback impact took place before the start of each session, typically three to four days after the previous session, so that responses didn't just reflect short-term effects.

> • Improvement was measured in four distinct clusters of symptoms -- cognitive function, fatigue, sleep and emotional well-being -- which were not highly connected at the start of the testing.

A follow-up study with a control group will provide a definitive answer, said Alvarez, who added that she hoped any future studies would involve a larger, more diverse population of cancer survivors, and incorporate pre- and post-functional MRI and neuropsychological tests that would confirm the study's findings.

She also hopes future studies will answer whether or not genetic markers exist that can help identify which people would benefit the most from neurofeedback and if neurofeedback would be able to keep chemo brain from emerging in the first place, if given in conjunction with standard cancer treatment."

Stress and the Brain

Normal stress relies on two key hormones: *adrenaline (epinephrine)* and *cortisol*. Very simply stated, adrenaline works in the short term, while cortisol has large momentum and works in the long term. I say 'normal' because the 'stress response' IS normal; it is a necessary physiologic response to a stimulus, either real or perceived. Yes, the stress response can also be activated if your brain *perceives* danger or any kind of threat, whether real or imagined.

Normally, a stressor triggers the release of adrenaline from your adrenal glands into the bloodstream to prepare the body for action. As a result, your heart beats faster, you begin to sweat, your breath becomes shallower, you shunt blood from your organs to your extremities, and your senses become more acute, all to prepare to run or flee. This is the so-called *fight or flight* response to the stressor, and they are wonderful, necessary and short-term.

This is the key point: stress responses are supposed to be short term responses to immediate danger as a protective measure to avoid calamity. The problem lies in that we live in a world where lions and bears are attacking us constantly! The lion of getting the kids to school, completing a project, pleasing the boss, and meeting ever-pressing deadlines coupled with the bears of financial pressures and keeping up with the Joneses have never been more apparent than today's modern society. What was created to be an infrequent response to life-or-death situations has become daily survival in the concrete jungle of life.

In the chronic stress response, the Sympathetic nervous system is hyper-triggered causing blood pressures to rise, and all bodily functions deemed unnecessary for imminent survival to suppress. Brain function is impaired, inflammation increases; there is no need for a sex-drive, detoxification, or bowel function if a bear is chasing you, you just need enough blood to your legs to outrun your friend.

The effect of the stress hormones on the brain is survival oriented. The initial surge of adrenaline can make you feel good, hence, why some Type One individuals are addicted to stress. Just as your levels of adrenaline start coming down, so rises the amount of cortisol flowing through your veins. Moreover, cortisol has a much larger momentum and enduring response than adrenaline, which means that even though it builds up slowly, it also takes a long time to go back to normal. Worse, should you continually engage adrenaline stimulation, your levels of cortisol also increase.

> *"All my life, I always wanted to be somebody. Now I see that I should have been more specific."*
> -Lily Tomlin

The combination of the rise of cortisol and the decrease of adrenaline, come the nasty side-effects of the stress hormones. It is during this time in the cycle you can feel worse, energy tumbles, anxious, and you may begin to have negative thoughts. You only feel the negative effects of stress as your body is *stressing down* and progressing towards a more relaxed state. When you are building up on adrenaline, in effect *stressing up*, you might even be feeling good – this can be addictive (the *adrenaline rush* and the consequent *adrenaline crash)*.

Cortisol then, gets the bad reputation as being the stress hormone with all the negative effects. In reality, cortisol plays some very important parts in homeostasis, energy production and blood sugar regulation. Prolonged cortisol production is the problem as it throws the glucose balance off in the brain (its primary food source) and leads to inflammation through a pathway called a TH17 response.

In the very early stages, a chronic stress response will not produce many noticeable brain symptoms. Functional Medicine testing reveals an adrenal stress response that is "out of whack", a Neurological Exam will show obvious signs, a "Brain Map" with a functional EEG will reveal asymmetry, and a Kinesiology Exam may reveal hormone imbalances long before symptoms drive a patient to see a physician.

Subjectively, you will eventually begin to feel a bit down and tired, especially during those periods when you are *crashing down* from the adrenaline, but most people would still not say that they feel depressed. Also, you would start sleeping a bit less than usual, having difficulty sleeping and possible waking at night and having a harder time getting back to sleep or just not feeling quite as fresh when you wake up.

Over time, more damage to neurons continues. Stress starts to take its toll as the amount of stress hormones increase. This is largely person-dependent, but most people start having problems with their digestive system, headaches, toxicity issues due to suppressed pathways, sexual dysfunction, poor sleep and having more frequent dreams. Since stress depresses the immune system, people also tend to fall sick with infections more often.

The bottom line is that prolonged stress damages neuronal pathways that may lead to depression and anxiety disorders; but it is a problem in the brain. Depression, anxiety, panic attacks, hyperventilation, bouts of psychosis, etc. are frontal lobe issues. As the insidious buildup of inflammation disables the communication between the prefrontal cortex deeper brain centers, the deeper centers lose their CEO. The prefrontal cortex is the parent, the boss, the executive that is supposed to calm the instinctual centers lying in the archeocortex. Raw emotions stored in the amygdala, hormone balance supplied by the hippocampus and impulsive behavior from the midbrain left on their own without the parenting of the prefrontal cortex can be disastrous.

Physiology of Depression, Anxiety, OCD, Panic Attacks...

- Neuron death in the hippocampus has been implicated

- Neurogenesis (the birth of new neurons) may be necessary for recovery

- Neurogenesis happens continuously in the healthy adult brain with proper stimulation and fuel

- Most antidepressants require about 2-3 weeks to have an effect and do nothing for neurogenesis (re-growth of damaged pathways)

- Stress may diminish neurogenesis

- People under stress may sleep less than usual, produce less IGF (growth factors for healing), increase brain inflammation, and increase rate of neuronal degeneration
- Stress and brain inflammation speeds aging

At least certain parts of the brain continuously renew themselves; this is what is called neuroplasticity. Sleep seems to be fundamental for this renewal process---perhaps the greatest amount of neurogenesis happens during sleep.

Food Additives and the Feingold Diet

In the 1960's, Dr. Feingold began his work on linking diet with behavior back, particularly with what was then called Hyperactive Disorder. He believed that the conventional medicine's wisdom about this condition was not accurate. At that time most doctors believed that children would just outgrow hyperactivity and that it had nothing to do with diet. Feingold was a radical yet many parents using his diet with their hyperactive child became instant believers. His work is continued through the Feingold Association which suggests the following from their website (www.feingold.org):

"The Feingold Program eliminates these additives:

- Artificial (synthetic) coloring
- Artificial (synthetic) flavoring
- Aspartame (NutraSweet, an artificial sweetener)
- Artificial (synthetic) preservatives BHA, BHT, TBHQ

In the beginning (Stage One) of the Feingold Program, aspirin and some foods containing salicylates are eliminated. Salicylate is a group of chemicals related to aspirin. There are several kinds of salicylate, which plants make as a natural pesticide to protect themselves. Those that are eliminated are listed in the salicylate list which is included also in the Program Handbook (found under the organization's membership). Most people can eventually tolerate at least some of these salicylates.

You will notice this dietary program is often referred to as a *program* because fragrances and non-food items which contain the chemicals listed above are also eliminated.

Where do food dyes come from?

Those pretty colors that make the "fruit punch" red, the gelatin green and the oatmeal blue are made from petroleum (crude oil) which is also the source for gasoline.

You will find them on the ingredient labels, listed as "Yellow No. 5," "Red 40," "Blue #1," etc. The label may say "FD&C" before the number. That means "Food, Drug & Cosmetics." When you see a number listed as "D&C" in a product, such as "D&C Red #33" it means that this coloring is considered safe for medicine (drugs) and cosmetics, but not for food.

What are artificial flavorings?

They are combinations of many chemicals, both natural and synthetic. An artificial flavoring may be composed of hundreds of separate chemicals, and there is no restriction on what a company can use to flavor food.

One source for imitation vanilla flavoring (called "vanillin") is the waste product of paper mills. Some companies built factories next to the pulp mills to turn the undesirable by-product into imitation flavoring, widely used in many cookies, candies and other foods.

What are BHA, BHT and TBHQ?

Those initials stand for three major preservatives found in many foods, especially in the United States. Like the dyes, they are made from petroleum (crude oil). Often, they are not listed in the ingredients.

Without doubt the mightiest thought the mind can entertain is the thought of God.
-AW Tozer

These chemicals may be listed as "anti-oxidants" because they prevent the fats in foods from "oxidizing" or becoming rancid (spoiling). There are many natural, beneficial anti-oxidants, but they are much more expensive than the synthetic versions.

There are other undesirable food additives (MSG, sodium benzoate, nitrites, sulfites, to name a few) but most of the additives used in foods have not been found to be as big a problem as those listed above.

Food additives are not new

Artificial colors have been around for more than 100 years. (Originally they were made from coal tar oil.) And children have been eating artificially colored and flavored products for decades.

But then . . . most children ate these additives infrequently. They got an occasional lollipop from the bank or barber shop. Cotton candy was found at the circus. Jelly beans were given at Easter, orange cupcakes at Halloween and candy canes at Christmas.

Today . . . the typical child growing up in the United States is exposed to these powerful chemicals all day, every day.

What the child growing up in the U.S. in the 1940's got:	What the child growing up in the U.S. today gets:
White toothpaste	Multi-colored toothpaste, perhaps with sparkles
Oatmeal	Sea Treasures Instant Oatmeal (turns milk blue)
Corn flakes	Fruity Pebbles
Toast & butter, jam	Pop Tarts
Cocoa made with natural ingredients	Cocoa made with artificial flavoring, & some with dyes.
Whipped cream	Cool Whip
No vitamins (or perhaps cod liver oil)	Flintstone vitamins with coloring & flavoring
White powder or bad-tasting liquid medicine	Bright pink, bubble-gum flavored chewable or liquid medicine
Sample school lunch: Meat loaf, freshly made mashed potatoes, vegetable. Milk, cupcake made from scratch.	**Sample school lunch:** Highly processed foods loaded with synthetic additives, no vegetable. Chocolate milk with artificial flavor.
Sample school beverage: Water from the drinking fountain	**Sample school beverage:** Soft drink with artificial color, flavor, caffeine, aspartame, etc.

Candy in the classroom a few times a year at class parties.	Candy (with synthetic additives) given frequently.

(Please consider becoming am member of the Feingold organization at www.feingold.org)

Artificial Sweeteners

Even though I mentioned these in the above piece on additives, artificial sweeteners are so damaging to the brain that they deserve their own section, maybe even an entire book. I have long preached to my patients that I'd rather have them eat sugar (yes, even my cancer patients) than eat artificial sweeteners. Aspartame is possibly the most common of these deadly additives so we'll discuss it here.

An Aspartame molecule is essentially made up of three different components: two natural amino acids (aspartic acid and phenylalanine), and a methyl ester bond, which includes Methanol. The methanol is released from the aspartame compound within hours of consumption and begins traveling through the body via the blood. Once the methyl ester bond is broken, it liberates methyl alcohol or methanol (wood alcohol). The problem with methanol is that it is a toxin that easily passes through your blood-brain barrier and is converted into formaldehyde.

Formaldehyde is dangerous poison that is causing the brain damage. While many animals are able to detoxify methanol in the body, humans do not have this capability. Formaldehyde is a serious neurotoxin and carcinogen. According to the EPA, Methanol is considered a 'cumulative poison' which means is accumulates in the body over time because the liver cannot excrete it. The more you consume over time the more poisoning takes place.

Methanol itself is a toxin that destroys the specialized astrocytes that form the myelin sheath covering the nerves in the brain. When this nerve insulation is removed, nerve signals fail. This causes the demyelinating symptoms that are commonly seen in diseases like MS, ALS as well as migraines that can include bizarre and inconsistent visual field disruptions, strange upper motor neuron findings and peripheral neuralgias and degeneration.

The EPA has accepted that a limit of consumption of 7.8 mg/day is acceptable. But considering it took the appointment of Donald Rumsfeld, former board member of the drug company that manufactured Aspartame, to Ronald Reagan's cabinet for the FDA to immediately approve it for use in food (the very same day Rumsfeld was sworn in), one might want to check the research.

According to Woodrow Monte, Ph.D., R.D., director of the Food Science and Nutrition Laboratory at Arizona State University:

"When diet sodas and soft drinks, sweetened with aspartame, are used to replace fluid loss during exercise and physical exertion in hot climates, the intake of methanol can exceed 250 mg/day or 32 times the Environmental Protection Agency's recommended limit of consumption for this cumulative toxin."

Further, he states that due to the lack of a couple of key enzymes, humans are many times more sensitive to the toxic effects of methanol than animals. Therefore, tests of aspartame or methanol on animals do not accurately reflect the danger for humans.

"There are no human or mammalian studies to evaluate the possible mutagenic, teratogenic, or carcinogenic effects of chronic administration of methyl alcohol," he said.

How can you know you are getting too much Methanol? You may experience headaches, ear buzzing, dizziness, nausea, gastrointestinal disturbances, weakness, vertigo, chills, memory lapses, numbness and shooting pains in the extremities, behavioral disturbances, and neuritis. Another very well-known sign of methanol poisoning is vision problems.

It gets worse. One of the amino acids in aspartame, aspartic acid is capable of crossing your blood-brain barrier. Aspartic acid taken in its free form (unbound to other amino acids in whole proteins) significantly raises the blood plasma level of aspartate and glutamate. Easily crossing the blood-brain barrier, aspartate or glutamate kill certain neurons by allowing the influx of too much calcium into the cells. This influx triggers excessive amounts of free radicals, destroying cells. The neural cell damage that can be caused by excessive aspartate and glutamate is why they are referred to as "excitotoxins." They "excite" or stimulate the neural cells to death. There it attacks your brain cells, creating a form of cellular overstimulation called excitotoxicity, which can lead to cell death.

Artificial sweeteners may just be the single worst things that one can consume legally. They have been linked to every chronic neurological illness including: Multiple sclerosis (MS), ALS, hormonal problems, memory loss, epilepsy, hearing loss, Alzheimer's, dementia, brain lesions, and neuroendocrine disorders.

Excitotoxins

Excitotoxins are a group of chemicals that when ingested, damage the neurons. The most well-known excitotoxin would probably be MSG, an additive that enhances the flavor of food. Excitotoxicity occurs when receptors for the excitatory neurotransmitter glutamate are over-activated. Dr. Russell Blaylock, MD, author of the book "Excitotoxins - the taste that kills" states that excitotoxicity may be involved in spinal cord injury, stroke, traumatic brain injury, hearing loss (through noise overexposure or to toxicity) and in neurodegenerative diseases of the brain) such as multiple sclerosis, Alzheimer's disease, amyotrophic lateral sclerosis (ALS), and Parkinson's disease.

Excitotoxins are food additives that food producers use to stimulate taste centers in the brain for the purpose of creating an addiction (or at least an increased desire) for the product. Candy, snack food (Doritos have 4 different excitotoxins in its ingredients), Oriental dishes, and prepared meals are notorious for adding excitotoxins to stimulate the brain to desire more. It's legal and considered 'good business practice' by food manufacturers as sales increase.

An interesting article published in the Journal of Neurotoxicology entitled, Excitotoxins in foods, Olney JW, Department of Psychiatry, Washington University School of Medicine, stated, "Evidence is reviewed pertaining to excitatory neurotoxins (excitotoxins) encountered in human food supply. The most frequently encountered food excitotoxin is glutamate (Glu)

> *Here's what you need to keep in mind. You no longer have yesterday. You do not yet have tomorrow. You have only today. This is the day the Lord has made. Live in it.*
> *-Max Lucado*

which is commercially added to many foods despite evidence that it can freely penetrate certain brain regions and rapidly destroy neurons by hyper-activating the NMDA subtype of Glu receptor. Hypersensitivity of NMDA receptors during development makes the immature nervous system especially sensitive to Glu excitotoxicity. On the other hand, elderly consumers are particularly sensitive to domoic acid, a powerful excitotoxic Glu analog that activates both NMDA and non-NMDA receptors. A high content of domoic acid in shell fish caused a recent food poisoning incident that killed some elderly victims and caused brain damage and memory impairment in others. Neurolathyrism is a crippling neurodegenerative condition associated with ingestion of a legume that naturally contains BOAA, an excitotoxic Glu analog that hyper-activates non-NMDA receptors. Thus, the human food supply is a source of excitotoxins that can damage the brain by one type of mechanism to which immature consumers are hyper-vulnerable, or by other mechanisms to which adult and elderly consumers are peculiarly sensitive."

Names of ingredients in foods that are excitotoxic:

Glutamic acid
Glutamate
Monosodium glutamate
Monopotassium glutamate
Calcium glutamate
Monoammonium glutamate
Magnesium glutamate
Natrium glutamate
Yeast extract
Anything "hydrolyzed"
Any "hydrolyzed protein"
Calcium caseinate,
Sodium caseinate

The following work synergistically with MSG to enhance flavor. If they are present for flavoring, so is MSG even if it is not listed:

Disodium 5'-guanylate
Disodium 5'-inosinate
Disodium 5'-ribonucleotides

Here's what Sally Fallon has to say about the health effects of MSG, in her book, "Dirty Secrets of the Food Processing Industry":

"While the industry was adding MSG to food in larger and larger amounts, in 1957 scientists found that mice became blind and obese when MSG was administered by feeding tube. In 1969, MSG-induced lesions were found in the hypothalamus region of the mouse brain. Subsequent studies pointed in the same direction. MSG is a neurotoxic substance that causes a wide range of reactions in humans, from temporary headaches to permanent brain damage. It is also associated with violent behavior. We have had a huge increase in Alzheimer's, brain cancer, seizures, multiple sclerosis and diseases of the nervous system, and one of the chief culprits is the flavorings in our food.

Ninety-five percent of processed foods contain MSG, and, in the late 1950s, it was even added to baby food. Manufacturers say they have voluntarily taken it out of the baby food, but they didn't really remove it; they just called it "hydrolyzed protein" instead.

An excellent book, *Excitotoxins*, by Russell Blaylock, describes how nerve cells either disintegrate or shrivel up in the presence of free glutamic acid if it gets past the blood-brain barrier. The glutamates in MSG are absorbed directly from the mouth to the brain. Some investigators believe that the great increase in violence in this country starting in

1960 is due to the increased use of MSG beginning in the late 1950s, particularly as it was added to baby foods."

Remember: By food industry definition, all MSG is "naturally occurring." "Natural" doesn't mean "safe." "Natural" only means that the ingredient started out in nature, like arsenic and hydrochloric acid.

When you eat real, whole foods, you automatically avoid MSG, aspartame and other excitotoxins. No need to memorize the whole list of different food additives, simply skip the processed junk and EAT REAL FOOD!"

The best advice is to eat food as close to the way God originally created it!

The Immune System and Antigen Responses

Autoimmune diseases in general are commonly overlooked in both traditional medicine and alternative healthcare. This is at least in part due to the fact that neither traditional medicine nor the alternative model of care has had much, if any, success in treating them. If we look at the traditional model of care, we find that complete immune suppression is the treatment of choice; its success rate is horrible and the patient is often killed by the medications meant to help them. Alternative solutions have fared better only as far as they didn't kill the patient.

Success is too often measured by the suppression of symptoms not correcting the cause that is producing an effect. The population seems to be okay with this model: Give my symptoms a name and then drug them into oblivion. Unfortunately, we are going to discover that this type of mentality is leading us down the road of destruction. The question they really need to ask is why they became sick in the first place. The answer to this question for many suffering people may lie in the fact that they have an immune destruction against their tissue that, unless stopped, is continuously progressing and may ultimately cause death. We cannot be satisfied with symptom suppression while ignoring the cause; we must never settle for a treatment that does not address the reason the disease exists; and we must become our own advocates, studying and demanding that our healthcare practitioner 'proves' their cure with logical understanding of the process itself.

The autoimmune response is an inflammatory response, which produces chemicals called cytokines, which are part of the body's natural defense system against outside invaders. The body's immune system may be separated into a Th1 and a Th2 response. The Th1 response may be thought of as the police force, the body's initial strike force against an invader or what is called an antigen. When an antigen is present, the Th1 system fires and kills the virus; should the bug be of a nasty persuasion and strong enough to resist the Th1 response, the Th2 system kicks in, creates antibodies against the virus, tagging them so appropriate white blood cells can finish them off. A person with an autoimmune disease has this process stuck in the 'on' position, either hyper-Th1 or hyper-Th2, which prolonged, destroys the tissue where the antigen is recognized. In the case of an antigen causing inflammation in the brain, it is equivalent to one's brain literally being on fire!

My opinion is that all chronic health patients should be tested for autoimmune disease. If the testing reveals such an attack, the battle is to figure out a way to dampen their immune activity. That is why it's necessary to do all the testing and select the most sensitive tests. "My doctor already tested me for gluten and he said it's not positive…" "But I had a H. pylori test already…" The blood test for gluten and H pylori are highly unreliable and reveal a lot of false negatives. You need to do the specialized stool and gene profile for gluten and the Urea Breathe Test for H. Pylori. New, more sensitive testing is being developed all the time; find a functional medicine doctor who is spending the time it takes to keep up on current trends. Immune panels need to be run with their Th1/Th2 cytokine breakdowns, a complete CBC with 1, 25 Vitamin D and 25 Vitamin D testing; get Homocystene levels, B-12 and a lipid panel. Always keep on digging and search for every possible antigen – there is often more than one!

> *"Thimerosol is the preservative in immunization shots, so anytime you get an immunization shot you are undergoing the same procedure that in the University Lab we used to give animals auto-immune disease-- -give a little tiny injection of mercury. And when you get an immunization shot you are getting a little tiny dose of mercury there."---*
> *Hal Huggins DDS*

TH1 and TH2 Balancing

There are 2 parts of your immune system, the TH1 and TH2 response. When a person is Auto-Immune, one of these systems is "hyper-firing" or Dominant. Balancing this system goes far in reducing a patient's symptoms:

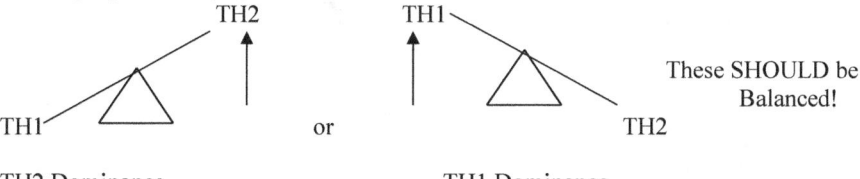

TH2 Dominance   TH1 Dominance

These SHOULD be Balanced!

There are specific dietary changes and supplements that can help and hinder the above response:
NOTE: ALL AI cases need Vitamin D, Glutathione, and Omega 3 fish oils +

Things that stimulate the TH1 response: (Take these if you are TH2 Dominant)
- Echinacea

- Goldenseal
- Garlic
- Vitamin C
- Any "Immune stimulants"
- Licorice root (Glycyrrhiza)
- Astragalus
- Eleuthero root
- Pau D'Arco
- Cat's Claw
- Beta-glucans, Maitake, Reishi and most other mushrooms
- Lemon Balm (Melissa officinalis)

Things that stimulate the TH2 response: (Take these if you are TH1 Dominant)
- Caffeine
- Green Tea (though it decreases IL-6 and is therefore beneficial)
- Grape Seed Extract
- Herbal barks (Cramp Bark, Pine Bark, and White Willow Bark)
- Lycopene
- Resveratrol
- Pycnogenol

Therefore, if a patient is TH1 Dominant, they should AVOID TH1 Stimulants and TAKE TH2 Stimulants

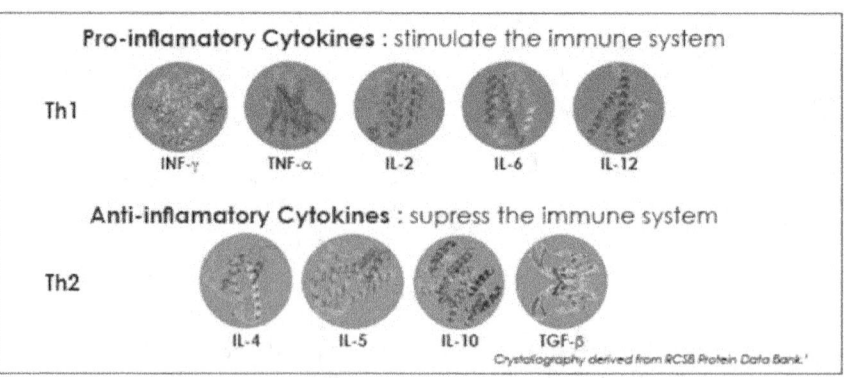

If one thinks that a child is sensitive to sugar, then one might attempt a no sugar diet for a couple of months. A no sugar diet avoids sugar, corn syrup, fructose, dextrose, honey, and maple syrup. The child's symptoms may increase for the first few days without sugar. Then reintroduce sugar and observe their behavior before and after. Even if a child were not sensitive to sugar one would want to keep their consumption of sugar low. Foods that are high in sugar are usually low in important essential nutrients, as well as usually contain artificial colors and flavors, chocolate, and saturated, hydrogenated and partially hydrogenated fats. In addition, if a child eats a large amount of sugar containing foods, this reduces their intake of high-density nutritious foods. Some suggestions to help avoid sugar in the diet: substitute all – fruit juices, fruit drinks or punches, with 100 percent unsweetened orange, grape, grapefruit or tomato juice. One should choose frozen and canned unsweetened fruits and pure fruit juices as well as fresh fruits for desserts and use small amounts of all fruit jams. A nutritious breakfast should include high protein food (eggs, homemade sausage, fresh fruit, gluten-free cereal or bread and raw milk). Most western children start the day with sugary cereal. Not only are these products high in sugar content, they also contain artificial colors and preservatives, which can all cause adverse reactions.

> *"A wise woman puts a grain of sugar into everything she says to a man, and takes a grain of salt with everything he says to her."*
> *-Helen Rowland quotes (English-American writer, 1876-1950)*

Yeast, Fungus and Mold

Yeasts are single-cell living organisms that are neither animal nor vegetable. They live on the surfaces of all living things, including fruits, vegetables, grains and your skin. They're part of the "microflora" which contributes in various ways to the health of their host with which they normally have a symbiotic relationship. Yeast itself is nutritious and small amounts of yeast gives bread its good yeasty taste. Yeast is a kind of fungus. Mildew, mold, mushrooms, monilia and candida are all names that are used to describe different types of yeast.

Candida albicans is normal in human flora and usually harmless living on the inner warm creases and crevices of the digestive tract and vagina. When your immune system is strong, candida yeasts cause no problems. But when you take broad-spectrum antibiotics for such conditions as acne, respiratory infections or cystitis (bladder infection), these drugs knock out friendly germs while they're knocking out enemies. Even overgrowth usually does not produce difficulty in a healthy child with a properly functioning brain and immune system. However, chronic use of antibiotics provides a less than optimum environment for both bacteria normally present and necessary for effective digestion and leads to mutant forms of the organisms.

Normal bacteria not only aid in digestion, but also create a certain pH of the intestine that helps suppress the growth of pathogens. When the bacteria are suppressed, the yeast can grow unchecked and Candida albicans is therefore thought to play a role in a number of health problems. These include recurrent infection, fatigue, irritability, hyperactivity, and other neurological symptoms, like short attention span, brain fog, and depression. It is also possible that some of these symptoms will also reflect a decrease in brain activation, especially of the left hemisphere that may be the prime cause of or be associated with other diseases or disorders co-existing with the yeast infection.

Valley Fever (Coccidioidomycosis [kok-sid-e-oy-do-my-co-sis] or "cocci" for short) is an infection of the lungs caused by a fungus that grows in the soil in the southern and central portions of California and the portions of Nevada, Arizona, New Mexico, Texas, and Utah. Valley Fever is also found in parts of Mexico, Central and South America.

Forty percent of people who are infected will develop symptoms such as cough, fever, exhaustion, rash, chest pain, night sweats, joint pain, muscle aches, headaches, weight loss, and lack of appetite. Some symptoms can last for weeks or even months and it can become chronic, lasting years and affecting neural centers, in a small percentage of people. Some people may develop severe disease infection outside the lungs or chronic symptoms. Certain groups of people are at higher risk of developing severe disease. In 2012, 12,920 cases of Valley Fever were reported to the Arizona Department of Health Services.

Mold is a nasty toxin in the body. In my experience, it's as hard to get rid of as chronic Lyme. The trichothecene mycotoxins produced by toxic black mold are neurotoxic. This means they can kill neurons in the brain and impair a person's mental ability. They also cause nervous disorders such as tremors and can cause personality changes such as mood swings and irritability.

Mold expert Dr. Jack Thrasher, estimates that as many as 40 percent of American schools and 25 percent of homes have mold infestations, unbeknownst to the people occupying those buildings. It follows that adverse health effects of mold may be reaching pandemic levels. Growing right along with mold are what are called "gram negative" and "gram positive" bacteria. Just like mold, they require moisture and organic material to thrive and are often found growing in the same places as mold, and the synergistic action between mold and bacteria further worsen inflammatory health conditions. Oftentimes, bacterial infections occur alongside fungal infections and make treatment more complicated.

According to Dr. Mercola, "Everyone is potentially at risk for toxic mold exposure, regardless of your geographic region, climate, socioeconomic status, race, age or gender. As with most other medical challenges, knowledge is your most powerful weapon. Scientific research has been emerging that connects mold exposure with various health conditions for which the causes were previously unknown. For example, in 2010, Fisk et al published a meta-analysis showing a substantially significant association between residential dampness and mold with respiratory infections and bronchitis."

A toxic exposure often impairs brain function but more importantly, it is usually exposure over time (prolonged, chronic and often unknown contact) that causes the greatest problem. Symptoms are varied and often unidentified. It's easy for someone to feel "crazy" rather than injured. An article titled "Psychological, Neuropsychological, and Electrocortical Effects of Mixed Mold Exposure" explains some of the implications of a toxic mold exposure.

The study stated, "The pattern of deficits commonly seen in mild traumatic brain injury is very similar to that found in mold-exposed individuals. This phenomenon--clinically referred to as 'brain fog'--is also common in individuals who suffer from multiple chemical sensitivities. Patients reported a loss of their sense of self, of their usual ways of doing things, and even of their personality. They were painfully aware of their deficits and were constantly frustrated by their loss of cognitive efficiency and frequent mistakes. This can be understood as a disturbance or dysfunction of the frontal cortical areas, as implicated in the QEEG findings and the relationship of exposure data to test performance in this study."

"Patients--including multiple family members--exposed to toxic molds reported moderate to severe levels of psychological distress related to the development of a wide range of physical, cognitive, and emotional symptoms. Problems included the frustration of trying to find knowledgeable and appropriate medical care, interference with social and work life, temporary or permanent abandonment of homes and possessions, financial stress, and anxiety and helplessness as a result of continuing poor health. Most of these patients, in absence of any significant premorbid psychiatric problems, could be diagnosed as suffering from acute stress, adjustment disorder, or post-traumatic stress."

Heavy Metal and other Environmental Toxins

There are many heavy metals in our environment both naturally and from pollution. The term "heavy metal" applies to a group of metals with similar chemical properties. Some of these, including copper, iron and zinc, play important roles in our bodies. Others have no known benefit for health.

Examples of these are lead, which is found in paint in old homes as well as many other sources; arsenic, which can be found in well water and wood products; and mercury, which can build up in fish that we eat.

Vaccinations

Here is an example of the inhumanity committed by these pharmaceutical companies regarding the vaccine Gardasil, marketed to young girls. All clinical trials of the vaccines to get it approved were done on children aged 15 and above, despite them currently being marketed for 9-year-olds. So far, 15,037 girls have reported adverse side effects from Gardasil alone to the Vaccine Adverse Event Reporting System (VAERS), and this number only reflects parents who underwent the hurdles required for reporting adverse reactions; one could safely multiply that by several. At the time of writing, 44 girls are officially known to have died from these vaccines. I'll guarantee you that if one person died from eating this book, it would be pulled off the market and I'd go to jail. The reported side effects include Guillian Barré Syndrome (paralysis lasting for years, or permanently — sometimes eventually causing suffocation), lupus, seizures, blood clots, and brain inflammation. Parents are usually not made aware of these risks.

In an article reported by Brent Lambert, July 2013, "Although these two vaccines are marketed as protection against cervical cancer, this claim is purely hypothetical. Studies have proven "there is no demonstrated relationship between the condition being vaccinated for and the rare cancers that the vaccine might prevent, but it is marketed to do that nonetheless. In fact, there is no actual evidence that the vaccine can prevent any cancer. From the manufacturers own admissions, the vaccine only works on 4 strains out of 40 for a specific venereal disease that dies on its own in a relatively short period, so the chance of it actually helping an individual is about the same as the chance of her being struck by a meteorite."

But vaccines are good for you, right? Let's reason together for a minute. Let us pretend that they are not made from aborted fetal tissue, do not contain any toxic metals, do not use formaldehyde, and don't have MSG and numerous other toxic chemicals. Let's pretend they are made from pure angel dust.

The reason someone would ever be vaccinated is to achieve immunity – protection from the disease. How does one become immune to a disease? First, there is no such thing as perfect immunity. If I had Chicken Pox as a child, I may or may not be immune to Chicken Pox later in life because when I did have it, my immune system fired a TH1 and then a TH2 reaction. A TH1 reaction is the killer cell side that attempts to destroy the pathogen. Should the disease process continue, the TH1 side of my immune response suppresses and my TH2 side fires to make antibodies. This is the key!

If my body has circulating antibodies from a particular pathogen it could be said that I have a relative immunity against that pathogen. I say 'relative immunity' because it depends on the number of antibodies that I have and the ferocity of pathogen that I may be exposed to. This is why most people (but not all) who had Chicken Pox as a child will not get Chicken Pox later in life should they be re-exposed.

So how does a vaccination work? If we could expose you with our imaginary angel dust vaccine that had just enough of the disease to fire a TH1 then a TH2 reaction that would cause you to create antibodies against the disease without creating a full-blown disease, then, and ONLY then would the vaccination result in immunity.

This is exactly why 47 children in my daughter's grade school last year were home sick with Chicken Pox and EVERY one of them previously were vaccinated against Chicken Pox! What the heck? How did that happen? Now you can explain it to your friends. Tell them, "It's simple really, if the vaccination didn't fire a TH1 then a TH2 reaction, your child will NOT create antibodies and they will NOT be immune. What Kool-Aid have you been drinking?" (You may want to leave that last part out)

In real life, vaccines are not made out of angel dust. Brain inflammation, Fibromyalgia, Chronic Fatigue, Depression, Anxiety, Autism, Cancer and other ASD disorders are linked to vaccination exposure. Does that mean that everyone getting vaccinated will have problems? Of course not; it depends on the individual's health of their liver and strength of their detoxification pathways. But to say that vaccines are innocuous and surety against contracting a disease is ludicrous.

I'll say nothing more about vaccinations; do your due diligence when making decisions that will affect you and your children for a lifetime.

This may help your Doctor

This section gets a bit more 'wordy' but may help your doctor if he/she isn't up on such data. Understanding the brain's immune response is crucial in helping patients with brain problems. Medicine's desire to medicate patients may quickly get them out of the office, placate the school, and even numb the symptoms but this practice is slowly eroding or culture and creating a dependency on the pharmacy. But that's really the purpose.

"For industry, every day a drug is held up from being marketed, represents a loss of 1 million to 2 million dollars of profit. The incentive is to review and approve the drugs as quickly as possible, and not stand in the way of profit-making. The FDA cooperates with that mandate." - David Graham, MD Neurologist, Associate Director for Science & Medicine, Office of Drug Safety, U.S. Food & Drug Administration *Employed by FDA for over twenty years*

In our opinion, the key to getting patients better, regardless of their symptoms is to figure out WHY they have this problem and know, and be able to test for, exactly WHAT is going to be best to heal it. I understand that is an overly simplified statement and every doctor would say, "Duh, that's what we're trying to do." However, understanding HOW to actually figure this stuff out gets a bit more complicated. After a concert pianist finished a concert, a spectator approached him and said, "You were fantastic, I want to be able to play the piano like you." Much to his surprise, the pianist retorted, "No you don't. If you did, you'd be home practicing 15 hours each day for the past 25 years," impressing the truth that there lies a grand chiasm between wanting to be an expert and willing to become one.

The original notion that the brain was an "immune-privileged" organ lacking the capability to produce an inflammatory response to an injury is no longer plausible.

Accumulated evidence during the last decade has shown that the CNS can mount a well-defined inflammatory response to a variety of insults including trauma, ischemia, transplantation, viral infections, toxins as well as neurodegenerative processes. New concepts are rapidly emerging as to the molecular mechanisms associated with the development of brain injury. In particular, the importance of cytokines, as well as adhesion molecules, has been emphasized in the propagation and maintenance of a CNS inflammatory response.

Virtually all brain based problems involve inflammation. Patients will be found to exhibit increased peripheral blood inflammatory biomarkers, including inflammatory cytokines, which have been shown to access the brain exogenously as well. Cytokines interact with virtually every pathophysiologic domain known to be involved in all the brain disorders, including neurotransmitter metabolism, neuroendocrine function, and neural plasticity.

Cytokines communicate and create effects in three ways: Autocrine, within the cell that creates it; paracrine, between cells; and endocrine, at a distance. Different cytokines have different functions which are all 'good', meaning they have a beneficial purpose. The problems arise when we see either prolonged secretion that becomes destructive or when the immune system has 'turned-on' against something that it can never kill.

So an example of the former would be a Chronic Lyme patient with an immune system attempting to kill a biotoxin (a living organism that normally should be able to be killed). However, in chronic biotoxin disorders, what makes them chronic is the fact that the immune system is unable to kill them for several reasons that we won't address in detail now. (Some bugs have the ability to hide within the cell and disable cellular markers that should normally clue an immune response to such infiltration – thereby staying 'ou-of-reach' from an immune response.)

An example of the later would be an immune response against mercury toxicity. The immune system should never have instigated an attack against mercury because remember, the immune system does one thing - it kills things. However, for a variety of reasons, this can happen and when it does, the patient will have a chronic, ramped-up immune response wherever the antigen is found.

As cytokines are classified, we separate them into groups. Chemicals typically found in a TH1 response are IL-1, IL-2, IL-8, IL-12, IL-18, IFN-gamma, TNF-alpha, and others. Those found in TH2 responses include IL-4, IL-5, IL-6, IL-10, IL-13, TGF-beta, and Fractalkine. But then we can separate cytokines into either PRO inflammatory (IL-1 alpha and beta, IL-2, IL-6, IL-8, IL-12, IL-18, IFN-gamma, NFkB, and TNF-alpha,) and ANTI inflammatory (IL-10, IL-13, TGF-beta, and Fractalkine).

Cytokine functions:

1. Most are secreted by many immune and non-immune cells (endothelial cells, astrocytes, fibroblast, adipocytes)

2. One cytokine can stimulate release of others (cascading effect)

3. Single cytokine can have effect on a broad range of cell types

4. Great redundancy-many cytokines can have same effect cytokine can stimulate release of others (cascading effect)

5. Many are involved in non-immune functions-bone formation, uterine function, endothelial cell function, etc.

6. Effect depends on timing: IL-6 acutely is protective and chronically is destructive

The cytokine 'tumor necrosis factor' (TNF-alpha) plays a significant role in brain immune and inflammatory activities. TNF-alpha is produced in the brain by microglial cells and astrocytes in response to various pathological processes such as biotoxin infiltration, ischemia, and trauma. Expect to have TNF-alpha increased excessively in Chronic Lyme disease (CLD), H-pylori infections, and chronic mold. Think of using supplementation like Green Tea Extract (EGCG) which has been proven to decrease TNF-alpha concentrations.

An example of function differentiation would be with NFkB. NFkB activation in microglial cells increases neuronal death but increases in the neuron itself are protective. Patients with MS see high levels of NFkB in the microglia near the plaque formation. Of course you want to figure out WHY this is happening but using products like Curcumin, Quercetin, Kaempferol, DHA, Green tea extract (EGCG), N-acetyl-L-cysteine, Silymarin, Selenium, Ginkgo biloba, Indole-3 , and Vitamin A (retinol).

NFkB is found in all cell types and has a variety of functions; many that you would not wish to be increased in chronic disorders. It also stimulates several other inflammatory cytokines like IL-6 (very destructive in chronic conditions) and TNFalpha.

A word about IL-6, a TH2, proinflammatory cytokine that is often elevated in cancer and other chronic infections like Lyme: IL-6 increases osteoclastic activity. Therefore, it inhibits bone healing; it is my opinion that one should take steps to decrease IL-6 levels and just assume they are high in all chronic disorders. Osteopenia, Osteoporosis, athletes with stress fractures, cancer patients with bone metastasis, and anyone with brain inflammation should consider steps to decrease IL-6 levels. What will do this? There currently is no medication. The only thing known, through a multitude of trails, to decrease IL-6 is Green Tea Extract (EGCG) and I typically recommend 1500-3000mg/day.

Other benefits of EGCGs: suppresses NFkB, decreases TNF-alpha, it is a chain-breaking antioxidant, Inhibits COX-1 and COX-2, Increases PPARs (peroxisome proliferator activated receptor), and Increases NAG-1. These are all huge positives for decreasing brain inflammation!

IFN-gamma primes macrophages and influences B cells (the TH2 system) to produce IgG (antibodies); TNF-alpha activates primes macrophages and Natural Killer (NK) cells to help pursue an immune assault. IL-2 is a growth factor that helps stimulate NK cells and causes Killer T-cells to proliferate; IL-4 is a growth factor for B cells and influences switch to IgE (an immediate response).

Dementias like Alzheimer's have been exhaustively been studied revealing a spike in certain cytokines (IL-1α, IL-2, IL-6, IL-12, TNF-α) with a high percentage of patients exhibiting autoantibodies to brain, meaning it often becomes an autoimmune disorder. IL-1alpha is an acute phase cytokine in the CNS that is commonly expressed within hours after a head injury but present in Alzheimer's. Microglial activation in these dementias are 6X higher than normal exhibiting numerous excessive, destructive cytokines and chemokines.

Studies injecting IFN- gamma produces depression, irritability, anxiety, low mood, cognitive impairment, apathy, loss of appetite and mild to severe fatigue. Depressed patients exhibit elevated IL-6 and IL-10 as well as acute phase proteins - haptoglobin and CRP.

Other nutrients that are known to reduce microglial activation that you may consider: Hesperidin, kaempferol, Magnesium, Quercetin, Curcumin, Ginseng, Luteolin, Anthocyanidins, Silymarin, DHA, Resveratrol, Consider

Curcumin is an excellent choice and has been shown to: Decreases reactive oxygen and nitrogen species (ROS and RNS), reduces microglial activation, decrease IL-12 production by macrophages and microglia, initiate a Th1 to Th2 shift, and reduce eicosanoid activation: LOX and COX.

But for right now, until that completeness, we have three things to do to lead us toward that consummation: Trust steadily in God, hope unswervingly, love extravagantly. And the best of the three is love.

Quercetin also inhibits NFkB, decreases nitric oxide (NO) production and suppresses inducible nitric oxide synthase (iNOS), potently inhibits 5-LOX and 12-LOX, inhibits proinflammatory cytokines (Th1), and Inhibits PLA2 as well as TNFalpha.

Vitamin D3 can be helpful and should be considered. My opinion is to test it and keep levels of at least 60. It has been shown to inhibit IL-12, IL-2, IFN-g and TNF-a, and decrease production of Th1 associated cytokines.

Silymarin (Milk thistle) also decreases production of NFkB, is a strong antioxidant that significantly reduces LPS induced TNF-alpha. It also inhibits JNK and MAPK p38 and increases cellular glutathione and SOD.

Fish Oil (omega-3 oils) will be discussed later but they are excellent fighters of brain inflammation, significantly decreasing IL-6, IL-10, IL-12 and TNF-alpha, decreases microglial activation and stimulates PPARs. Vitamin A (Retinols) also inhibit NFkB activation, increase TGF-beta, decrease TNF-alpha, and decrease iNOS.

Vitamin E (beta and gamma tocotrienols – not alpha) suppresses IL-6, IL-10, IL-12, and TNF-alpha, suppresses inflammatory eicosanoids, and when added to N-3 oils (fish oils) further lowering of these cytokines occurs. Ginkgo biloba inhibits NFkB activation by lipopolysaccharide, and reduces TNF-a stimulation by LPS.

These other nutrients have shown that they reduce microglial activation: Hesperidin, Kaempferol, Magnesium, Quercetin, Curcumin, Ginseng, Luteolin, Anthocyanidins, Silymarin, DHA, and Resveratrol.

Farooqu and Horrocks (2001) reporting in the Journal of Molecular Neuroscience, state that plasmalogens are glycerol-phospholipids of neural membranes, rate-limiting enzymes, are in the peroxisomes and are induced by docosahexaenoic acid (DHA). The authors suggest that deficiencies of DHA and plasmalogens occur in peroxisomal disorders, like Alzheimer's disease, depression, and ADHD, The authors claim that this situation may be responsible for abnormal signal transduction associated with learning disability, cognitive deficit, and visual dysfunction. These abnormalities in the signal-transduction process can be partially corrected by supplementation with a diet enriched with DHA or essential fatty acids.

The symptoms of essential fatty acid deficiencies include:

- Excessive thirst
- Frequent urination
- Dry skin
- Dry hair
- Dandruff
- Soft and brittle nails
- Small hard little white bumps on the backs of the arms, elbows or thighs.

There are two essential fatty acids relevant to our discussion: linolenic acid, an omega-6 fatty acid and alpha-linolenic acid, an omega-3 fatty acid. These are the precursor molecules for making long chain fatty acids such as dihommo-gamma-linolenic acid (DGLA), arachadonic acid, eccosapentaenoic acid (EPA) and docosahexaenoic acid (DHA). Omega-6 and Omega-3 fatty acids are essential because they help make up the cell membrane around every cell including brain cells. The balance of these essential fatty acids helps to determine the fluidity of the membrane and the ability of molecules to enter and exit the cell. This balance also affects the ability of molecules to bind to receptors in the membrane. These long chain fatty acids are also critical because the body converts them to prostaglandins and other important molecules that help cells communicate with each other. Arachadonic and DHA are more concentrated in the brain and retina than in other cells. They therefore play a crucial role in brain and nervous system function. Studies have suggested that approximately 40 percent of boys with ADHD have significantly lower levels of omega-3 and 6 fatty acids than controls with normal behavior (Mitchell et al., 1987). However, boys with ADHD have few symptoms of fatty acid deficiencies and have blood levels comparable to boys in the control group. It is thought that the reason for lower levels could include lower dietary intake or a metabolic block in the omega-3 and 6 fatty acid pathways.

Ways to increase intake of essential fatty acids, especially omega-3, is to use cold process cod liver oils or olive oils for homemade salad dressing. These oils can be included into spaghetti sauce, soup, etc. or used to make a pasta salad; also baking with them is good. Frying with these oils should be avoided because the molecules do not sustain their structure with high heat and oxygen so use coconut oil in frying at higher temperatures. Flaxseed oil is a more concentrated source of omega-6 and 9 fatty acids and therefore should be avoided. Beans are also a good source of essential fatty acids, especially navy and kidney. Tofu is soy and should be avoided. Cold water fish, like salmon, tuna, mackerel, and sardines are an excellent source of omega-3 fatty acids.

In some cases, a patient may have a genetic predisposition to a certain mineral or vitamin deficiency and therefore that individual may require supplementation to compensate for the inherited decrease in production, absorption, or inability to produce the relevant substances on their own. In these cases, the deficiencies may exacerbate the symptoms and even create additional symptoms. We like to run special testing when this is suspected that test measures intracellular nutrients. It is our opinion that nutrient blood testing that does NOT measure intracellular nutrients will not be accurate.

Nutrients and supplements that have been shown, under controlled circumstances, to enhance brain function and cognitive abilities and improve behavior need to be TESTED SPECIFICALLY as each case is completely different and I absolutely do NOT advocate a 'cookie cutter' approach!

Chapter Four

Treat the PROBLEM at BOTH Fronts

CAUSE OF BRAIN INFLAMMATION

A) Fixing the barriers

B) Finding and fixing the source

RESULTANT NEUROLOGICAL DEFICITS

C) Re-paving the damaged pathways

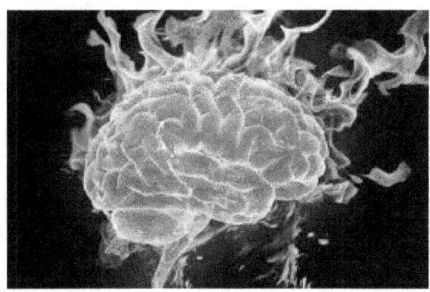

A. Fixing the Barriers

And the LORD said to Joshua: "See! I have given Jericho into your hand, its king, *and* the mighty men of valor. You shall march around the city, all *you* men of war; you shall go all around the city once. This you shall do six days. And seven priests shall bear seven trumpets of rams' horns before the ark. But the seventh day you shall march around the city seven times and the priests shall blow the trumpets. It shall come to pass, when they make a long *blast* with the ram's horn, *and* when you hear the sound of the trumpet, that all the people shall shout with a great shout; then the wall of the city will fall down flat. And the people shall go up every man straight before him."

In centuries past, the conquest of fortified cities posed a formidable problem for an attacking army, particularly if it was a "people's army" without specialized equipment. The adventure beginning with two Israelite spies in the house of Rahab as depicted in the Biblical book of Joshua details the strategic necessity of removing barriers.

"So the people shouted when *the priests* blew the trumpets. And it happened when the people heard the sound of the trumpet, and the people shouted with a great shout, that the wall fell down flat." Most read this account and believe that it was imply a miraculous work of God, one devoid of natural explanation. Miracles are usually explained this way and in so doing, we tend to wobble along the edge magic. Though many things our Creator has done have yet to be explained, I contend that He never has nor will either perform magic or break the physical laws that He created to uphold His universe.

That said, we have two options of explanation regarding Jericho

The fall of the walls of Jericho was indeed a wondrous event and the text properly sees God as the agent in the sense that it was He who inspired Joshua to come up with his ingenious plan

As stated in the previous chapters, a break in the barriers is what causes problems. Think of your skin; it is a barrier against infection that protects your body from the outside world. Should you cut your arm, a local immune response ensues to kill any possible infective pathogens from damaging the tissue, collagen fibers gather to heal the wound, growth factors (IGF-1) are released to stimulate rapid recovery until the barrier is rebuilt. This is exactly what happens in your gut barrier and your blood-brain barrier (also in your alveoli of your lung but we won't talk about that now).

If you decided to repeated slash your arm, the barrier is continually breached and pathogens will definitely enter the bloodstream. So it is with the rest of the barriers. Continual damage equals enemy entrance regardless of the gallant efforts of the kings guards attempting to protect the castle.

Healing the gut barrier should be the first intent of the practitioner. 2000 years ago Hippocrates said it well, "bad digestion is the root of all evil." More recently, Nobel laureate Elie Metchnikoff said: "Death begins in the colon." As I stated in the above chapters, every doctor must first check patients for hypochlorhydria (decreased HCl production) and supplement with HCl and digestive enzymes.

Compromise in the integrity of the gut barrier causes increase intestinal permeability, or Leaky Gut Syndrome (LGS), causing the tight junctions of the intestinal mucosa to become compromised. The space between the cells becomes widened and permeable so that large, undigested compounds, toxins and bacteria can pass through the intestinal mucosa and into the circulatory system.

The foreign compounds and organisms then react with the immune system which sees them as antigens (enemy invaders) that need to be broken down and destroyed. These antigens challenge the immune system and trigger the production of antibodies to neutralize the antigens which then begins a cycle of inflammation and self-cell damage.

The immune responses, resulting in the production of pro-inflammatory cytokines, are attempting to kill the foreign invaders and this is where we really have problems as many of the foreign invaders (antigens) are NOT living. What if protein particles (peptides) of food (like gluten) are the invaders that pass through the damaged gut wall?

Huge amounts of pro-inflammatory cytokines can flood the system to kill something that CANNOT BE KILLED leading to accelerated destruction of the GI tract cells themselves, other organs and tissues of the body, and (it gets worse), your Th2 response starts making antibodies against your OWN tissue. This is then, by definition, an autoimmune disease!

We spoke about what happens to the immune response when we get gut border damage, but what causes the damage? Below is a list of some of the things that can initially set this vicious cycle in motion and depending on the cause in your case, will dictate the treatment. By this I mean that if casein is a cause of inflammation, you must remove casein for the diet as well as taking the appropriate steps that I outline below if you are going to have success. I can't tell you how many patients have tried to circumvent this obvious fact because they refuse to change their diet. It's a bit like trying to rebuild the dike in the middle of Katrina – good luck with that.

- Gluten: In genetically pre-disposed people, a single dose of gluten, a dietary protein found in wheat, rye, spelt, barley, and malt can cause increased intestinal permeability.
- Casein: It is a protein found in large quantities in cow's milk.
- Fast Foods: Chemicals in processed foods are extremely irritating.
- Alcohol: Promotes intestinal bacterial growth and permeability.
- Antibiotics: Dramatically upset the intestinal environment.
- Cortico-Steroids: Decrease systemic immune reactions and cause all sorts of problems
- Antacids: They upset acid levels in the stomach necessary for good digestion.

- H Pylori: This extremely common bacteria is the major cause of gastric and duodenal ulcers, cancer, heart disease, and all endothelial damage.
- Intestinal Dysbiosis: This is a condition where microbial imbalances develop in the gut. In small amounts, microbial colonies found in the gut are usually benign or beneficial. When the balance is disturbed due to factors like antibiotic exposure or alcohol misuse, an overgrowth of one or more of the disturbed colonies can develop into a chronic and pervasive imbalance allowing pathogenic microbes to take control.
- Intestinal viruses, mold, Lyme, parasites, and other pathogens.
- Stress: Even normal life stress can predispose us to gut inflammation.
- Blood Sugar Imbalances: They can alter our stress response and trigger multiple pathways leading to leaky gut. Everyone should be tested for dysglycemia. Fasting (morning) blood sugars over 90 can lead to gut problems.
- Sleep disturbances: When we have a normal night sleep, our brain secretes IGF-1, a growth hormone that stimulate a Th1 response in the gut to kill off pathogens that may be present from the day. Poor sleep equals poor gut. We see this commonly with those on swing shift work schedules. This is also part of a common vicious cycle with cortisol, the hippocampus and glucose creation in the liver which we'll discuss when we talk about testing.
- Hormone Imbalances: They have a major influence on GI Function.
  - The thyroid hormones T4 and T3 have been shown to protect the intestinal mucosal lining from injury.
  - Low levels of T4 and T3 can cause decreased stimulation of gastric and intestinal cells leading to ulcers (from H. pylori infiltration not being killed by the HCl), intestinal permeability, decreased secretion of pancreatic enzymes, impair gall bladder function and decreased bowel motility.
  - Decreased HCL can allow parasites and bacteria to pass through the stomach into the intestines since proper pH of the stomach is the first line of defense against pathogens.
  - Proper levels of Estradiol decrease colonic permeability.
  - Progesterone protects the intestinal lining.
  - Lack of testosterone delays intestinal healing.

Increased cytokine and antibody production in turn, increases intestinal barrier permeability and a vicious cycle ensues due to an exaggerated immune response both within the gut and systemically. These very cytokines, circulating in the blood can then damage the blood-brain barrier even in the absence of circulating toxins!

Some Foods to avoid if you have Leaky Gut

- Remove all potentially irritating foods and potential allergens. Most common is gluten, casein (dairy), and soy but should you have a gluten sensitivity, it is common to have immune responses against gluten-like foods as well (chocolate, sesame, hemp, buckwheat, sorghum, millet, amaranth, quinoa, yeast, tapioca, oats, corn, rice, and potato)
- Processed Foods: including canned, boxed and bottled foods
- Sugars: including corn syrup, molasses, honey, chocolate, candy
- High Glycemic Fruits: like potatoes, watermelon, mango, pineapple and raisins
- All Grains: including wheat, oats, rice, soy, corn, wheat germ, quinoa (look up Paleo Diet)
- Gluten Containing Compounds: such as processed salad dressing, ketchup, soy sauce, barbecue sauces, mayonnaise, condiments and modified food starch
- Cow's milk products: including whey, cheeses, creams, yogurt
- Soy: including soy milk, soy sauce, soy protein, etc.
- Eggs
- Alcohol: including beer, wine, etc.
- Lectins: including nuts, beans, soy, potatoes, tomatoes, eggplant, peppers, peanut oil and soy oil

Foods to eat that can Help Leaky Gut

- Most Vegetables: except tomatoes, potatoes (sweet potatoes are okay) and mushrooms
- Fermented Foods: like sauerkraut, kimchi, pickled ginger, kombucha tea, homemade coconut yogurt and pickles
- Meats: including fish, chicken, beef, lamb, etc.
- Low Glycemic Fruits: including apricots, plums, apples, peaches, pears, cherries and berries
- Coconut: including fresh coconut, coconut oil, coconut milk
- Herbal teas, olives, olive oil

> *Learn from yesterday, live for today, hope for tomorrow. The important thing is not to stop questioning.*
> *Albert Einstein*

The following are some possible things to consider treating gut pathogens. However, we strongly suggest that you consult your doctor before attempting any protocols in this book. Again, this book is meant to be a guide for your doctor to test and treat your condition. Finding out WHY you have a barrier problem is essential in our mind and must not be overlooked. If your doctor doesn't know how to properly test may I suggest that you find another doctor? Rarely a week goes by that we don't have a doctor call our office asking to spend a week here to 'pick our brains'. Personally, I just don't have much left up there and this is one reason we put this book together and why we hole Clinicals in our office for practitioners. Have your doctor register under the "Doctors only" tab on our website for more in-depth information and details on implementing correction.

Yeast/Candida Intestinal Dysbiosis

- Undecylenic Acid
- Caprylic Acid
- Uva Ursi
- Cat's Claw
- Pau D'Arco

Parasites and other Pathogens

- Olive Leaf Extract
- Garlic Extract
- Wormwood
- Black Walnut
- Medicinal Mushrooms
- Nopal
- Rhubarb root
- Astragalus
- Echinacea
- Licorice root

H Pylori

- Golden Seal Root Extract
- Medicinal Mushrooms
- Oregano Oil Extract
- Barberry Extract
- Grapefruit Seed Extract
- Oregon Grape Root Extract
- Berberis Extract
- Coptis Chinensis Extract
- Yerba Mansa Extract

Intestinal Microbial Support

- Saccharomyces Boulardii
- Lactobacillus Sporogenes
- Lactobacilli Acidophilus
- Arabinogalactin

Restoration and Healthy Maintenance of the Intestinal Mucosa

- L-Glutamine
- Deglycyrrhizinated Licorice
- Aloe Leaf Extract
- Spanish Moss
- Marshmallow Extract
- Gamma Oryzanol
- Immunoglobulin G, A, M, D, and E
- IGF-1 and 2
- Transforming Growth Factors
- Transferrin
- Colostrum
- N-Acetyl Glucosamine
- Modified Citrus Pectin
- Slippery Elm herb
- Mucin
- Chamomile
- Okra Extract
- Cat's Claw herb
- MSM
- Quercetin
- Boswelia
- Proline-Rich Polypeptides

Gluten Sensitivity

Gluten Sensitivity is a systemic autoimmune disease attacking everywhere the gliadin peptides (protein particles) can be found. Gluten, a long-chain protein found in many grains is a key factor in most GI and autoimmune conditions. It has been said that the majority of the US population have undiagnosed Gluten Sensitivity. We FIRMLY believe, even if you test negative for gluten sensitivity, that all patients with brain-based issues REMOVE ALL GLUTEN FROM THEIR DIET. It is just too inflammatory!

So, it is essential to learn what foods contain gluten. I'll include a list below but I strongly suggest that you simply Google "gluten free diet" or "gluten free living" and you will get a plethora of information.

Gluten Containing Grains: Wheat, Spelt, Kamut, Oats (technically not a gluten, but usually gluten contaminated when not from gluten-free farms so you MUST eat only certified Gluten-free oats), Rye, and Barley.

Some Hidden Sources of Gluten: Soy Sauce, Food Starches, Food Emulsifiers, Artificial Food Colorings, Malt extract, flavor and syrup, Dextrins

Chronic Stress leads to a breakdown of immune tolerance.

Gluten Sensitivity Testing

For the most part, Gluten Sensitivity testing is insufficient and misses many cases of Gluten Sensitivity. Most lab testing, (whether it be blood, saliva or stool) measures only antibodies to Alpha-Gliadin (one specific component of wheat protein). However, wheat protein consists of other components, all of which have the capacity to challenge the immune system.

A new, state-of-the-art test from Cyrex Labs, measures immune reactions to 24 different components found in gluten-containing grains, including the de-aminated glutens found in processed wheat and wheat germ. Another Lab – EnteroLab measures genetic markers that are 'turned-on' with gluten sensitivity and can be helpful in diagnosing the entire family with one test.

If sensitivity to gluten or any of its components is discovered, total abstinence is necessary. The inflammatory responses to even a single portion of gluten, in a sensitive individual, can set forward a cascade of immunological reactions that can last upwards to eight months.

Once the gut barrier has been breached, enemies are circulating in the blood and can damage the next barrier – the vessel endothelial layer. The blood vessel's barrier is a single-celled intimal layer that has thousands of different receptors that 'turn-on" different functions and allow nutrients to pass.

Vascular injury can come from a near infinite number of sources. Chemical insult can come from Bio-toxins, Nutritional Toxins, and Metabolic Sterile Antigens (normal cellular waste). Bio-Mechanical insult can result from changes in hemodynamics (BP, Blood flow…). Any insult results in three possible outcomes: Local inflammation, Oxidative stress, or autoimmune dysfunction; all three of these are actually correct, though exaggerated responses attempting to heal the vessel wall.

We believe that though the patient may not need to understand the mechanisms involved, the doctor should become familiar with endothelial dysfunction to better think-through strategic methods of repair. So I'm going to bore you with a lot of cellular biology for a few pages.

Our Step-up program for healing the Barriers (and everything else)

In our office, healing barriers has become a priority. However, we've found that there exists a separation between that which patients *should* do and that which they are *willing* to do. This being true, we've developed a sort of hierarchy to healing the gut, which, if you read the list below, starts with the minimal approach a patient may choose and ends with the most radical. Understand that we typically don't explain these choices to our patients without giving them our best recommendation based on our clinical testing, but ultimately, the patient must choose the level of commitment which most assuredly reflects in their level of success.

1. Getting off of the 'standard American diet' (SAD). This means that the patient starts to make dietary changes as outlined in this book and eliminates artificial sweeteners, decreases sugar consumption, stops eating fast food, eats more organic food, and learns to read labels and become conscious of what they put into their mouth. Most of our patients have already passed this threshold before walking through our doors as they have been to countless doctors and read, studied, searched and attempted as many things as possible to achieve health. Honestly, if a sick person won't make these initial simple changes, the promise of health will elude them. We highly recommend the Weston A. Price Foundation for more information on what was originally intended as a diet for mankind. (see www.westonaprice.org)

2. Elimination of food sensitivities and inflammatory consumables. One need not even undergo expensive testing to determine food sensitivities as ill individuals can just presume they exist. Foods that patients choosing this second level must avoid include gluten (wheat, rye, spelt, malt, barley) and possibly dairy (though we do recommend raw dairy once gut healing has begun).

3. Going completely Paleo. A Paleo diet eliminates all grains due to their inflammatory nature. Though one may not need to stay "Paleo" forever, through the healing process, it is highly recommended. There are numerous books and websites that give the reader details in living this lifestyle.

4. The GAPS diet. Below you'll find our version of the GAPS diet that Dr. Natasha Campbell-McBride so eloquently explains in her book "Gut and Psychology Syndrome". This diet is high in the fat necessary to heal epithelial layers (the skin of both your insides and outsides).

5. Fecal transplantation. This is the most radical yet often life-saving approach to healing the gut barrier which we recommend yet beyond the scope of this book to discuss.

In our office, none of the above approaches are incorporated without testing, correcting causes, utilizing specific nutrients such as HCl, digestive enzymes, probiotics, etc. It is important to note that while this book may be used by a patient or doctor as a guideline of possible care paths, it is NOT a protocol. Personally, I abhor protocols as they lump patients into a die that was cast for the 'average'. People are individuals and must be treated as such.

Our 30 Day Intensive Immune-Barrier Recovery Dietary Program

this is our modification of the GAPS diet

30 Day Intensive Immune System Recovery Dietary Program

We strongly recommend that you follow the GAPS INTRODUCTION DIET for a full 30 days. You will start the diet on STAGE ONE and gradually move through the stages at your own pace, as tolerated by your body. Each stage will include a list of foods that you will be able to eat. You do not HAVE to eat all the foods that are in each stage, but you should not eat anything else other than what is listed for that particular stage.

Every morning, upon waking drink 1 cup of mineral or filtered water and take your **PROBIOTIC supplement**. Allow 30-60 minutes to pass before eating.
(You may also place another ¼ tsp of probiotic into a warm water enema or coffee enema. This is in addition to what you take orally.)

Allowed foods can also be purchased at www.farmmatch.com (beef, bones, raw kefir, raw yogurt, whey, etc).
While on this diet, be prepared to eat as often as you like, while your body adjusts to this super digestible food. The same foods can be served throughout the day to

minimize cooking and clean up.

Detoxification therapies - detox baths (see book for details), coffee enemas, filtered water intake, rebounding (jumping on mini-trampoline), infrared saunas.

FULL GAPS DIET
Although it is best and most healing to the body to complete the GAPS INTRODUCTION 30 day program, the FULL GAPS DIET can be started first for those that cannot complete the more restrictive INTRO diet.

The best foods in the FULLGAPS DIET are eggs (if tolerated), fresh meats (not preserved), fish, shellfish, fresh vegetables and fruit, nuts and seeds, garlic and olive oil. Apart from eating vegetables cooked, it is important to have some raw vegetables with meals, as they contain vital enzymes to assist digestion of the meats. Fruit should be eaten on their own, not with meals, as they have a very different digestion pattern and can make the work harder for the stomach. Fruit should be given as a snack between meals.

It is very important to have plenty of natural fats in every meal from meats, butter, ghee, coconut (if tolerated) and cold pressed olive oil. Animal fats on meats are particularly valuable. Fermented foods (sauerkraut, yogurt, and kefir) are also a very important part of this diet in addition to homemade meat or fish stock. It is recommended to take a cup of warm meat or fish stock with every meal as a drink as well as soups and stews made with the meat or fish stock. The stock, kefir and fermented vegetables will over time restore the stomach acid production, which will improve digestion.

It is best to avoid processed foods (any packet or tinned foods). They are stripped from most nutrients that were present in the fresh ingredients used for making these foods. They are a hard work for the digestive system and they damage the healthy gut flora balance. On top of that they usually contain a lot of artificial chemicals, detrimental to health, like preservatives, colorants, etc. Try to buy foods in the form that nature made them, as fresh as possible.

FOODS TO AVOID

All sugar substitutes, artificial sweeteners
Acidophilus milk
Agar-agar (a gelling agent)
Agave syrup - main carbohydrate is a complex form of fructose
Algae - can aggravate an already disturbed immune system
Aloe Vera – unless the Doctor tests you
Amaranth - is a grain substitute, contains starches
Apple juice - usually has sugar added during processing
Arrowroot - is a mucilaginous herb and loaded with starch
Baked beans

Baker's yeast - contains saccharamyces cerevisae
Baking powder and raising agents of all kind -
Balsamic vinegar - most found in stores have added sugar
Barley
Bean flour and sprouts
Bee pollen - irritating to a damaged gut
Beer – even gluten-free
Bhindi or okra
Bicarbonate of soda
Bitter Gourd
Black-eye beans
Bologna
Bouillon cubes or granules
Brandy
Buckwheat
Bulgur
Butter beans
Buttermilk
Canellini beans
Canned vegetables and fruit
Carob
Carrageenan - is seaweed and high in polysaccharides
Cellulose gum
Cereals, including all breakfast cereals
Cheeses – ALL that are NOT RAW
Chestnuts and chestnut flour
Chewing gum - contain sugars or sugar substitutes
Chick peas
Chickory root - contains high amounts of FOS
Chocolate
Cocoa powder - please see "FAQs" for more information
Coffee, instant and coffee substitutes
Cooking oils
Cordials
Corn – corn is a GRAIN
Cornstarch
Corn syrup
Cottonseed oil (not a food)
Couscous
Cream - contains lactose
Cream of Tartar
Dextrose
Fava beans
Fish that is preserved, smoked, salted, breaded and canned
Flour, made out of grains

FOS (fructooligosaccharides)
Fructose that is extracted from corn
Fruit that is canned or preserved
Garbanzo beans
Grains, all
Ham
Hot dogs
Ice-cream, commercial
Jams / Jellies
Jerusalem artichoke
Ketchup, commercially available
Lactose
Liqueurs
Margarines and butter replacements
Meats that are processed, preserved, smoked and salted
Millet
Milk from soy, rice, canned coconut milk
Milk, that is NOT raw or is dried
Molasses
Mungbeans
Nuts that are salted, roasted and coated
Oats – even gluten-free
Okra - mucilaginous food
Parsnips
Pasta, of any kind
Potato white or sweet
Quinoa - 60% starch
Rice – all – occasional WILD rice
Rye
Semolina
Sherry
Soda, soft drinks, pop is OUT
Sour cream, commercial
Soy unless fermented
Spelt
Starch
Sugar or sucrose of any kind
Tapioca - starch
Tea, instant
Triticale
Turkey loaf or other prepared meats
Vegetables, canned or preserved
Wheat, Wheat germ
Yams
Yogurt, commercial – buy RAW or make yourself

RECOMMENDED FOODS

Almonds, including almond butter and oil
Apples
Apricots, fresh or dried
Artichoke, French
Asiago cheese
Asparagus
Aubergine (eggplant)
Avocados, including avocado oil
Bananas (ripe only with brown spots on the skin)
Beans, dried white (navy), string beans and lima beans properly prepared
Beef, fresh or frozen
Beets or beetroot
Berries, all kinds
Black, white and red pepper: ground and pepper corns
Black radish
Blue cheese
Bok Choy
Brazil nuts
Brick cheese
Brie cheese
Broccoli
Brussels sprouts
Butter
Cabbage
Camembert cheese
Canned fish in oil or water only
Capers
Carrots
Cashew nuts, fresh only
Cauliflower
Cayenne pepper
Celeriac
Celery
Cellulose in supplements
Cheddar cheese
Cherimoya (custard apple or sharifa)
Cherries
Chicken, fresh or frozen
Cinnamon
Citric acid
Coconut, fresh or dried (shredded) without any additives
Coconut milk
Coconut oil
Coffee, weak and freshly made, not instant

Collard greens
Colby cheese
Courgette (zucchini)
Coriander, fresh or dried
Cucumber
Dates, fresh or dried without any additives (not soaked in syrup)
Dill, fresh or dried
Duck, fresh or frozen
Edam cheese
Eggplant (aubergine)
Eggs, fresh
Filberts
Fish, fresh or frozen, canned in its juice or oil
Game, fresh or frozen
Garlic
Ghee, homemade (many store varieties contain non-allowed ingredients)
Gin, occasionally
Ginger root, fresh
Goose, fresh or frozen
Gorgonzola cheese
Gouda cheese
Grapefruit
Grapes
Haricot beans, properly prepared
Havarti cheese
Hazelnuts
Herbal teas
Herbs, fresh or dried without additives
Honey, natural
Juices freshly pressed from permitted fruit and vegetables
Kale
Kiwi fruit
Kumquats
Lamb, fresh or frozen
Lemons
Lentils
Lettuce, all kinds
Lima beans (dried and fresh)
Limburger cheese
Limes
Mangoes
Meats, fresh or frozen
Melons
Monterey (Jack) cheese
Muenster cheese
Mushrooms

Mustard seeds, pure powder and gourmet types without any non-allowed ingredients
Nectarines
Nut flour or ground nuts (usually ground blanched almonds)
Nutmeg
Nuts, all kinds freshly shelled, not roasted, salted or coated (any roasting must be done at home)
Olive oil, virgin cold-pressed
Olives preserved without sugar or any other non-allowed ingredients
Onions
Oranges
Papayas
Parmesan cheese
Parsley
Peaches
Peanut butter, without additives
Peanuts, fresh or roasted in their shells
Pears
Peas, dried split and fresh green
Pecans
Peppers (green, yellow, red, and orange)
Pheasant, fresh or frozen
Pickles, without sugar or any other non-allowed ingredients
Pigeon, fresh or frozen
Pineapples, fresh
Pork, fresh or frozen
Port du Salut cheese
Poultry, fresh or frozen
Prunes, dried without any additives or in their own juice
Pumpkin
Quail, fresh or frozen
Raisins
Rhubarb
Roquefort cheese
Romano cheese
Satsumas
Scotch, occasionally
Seaweed fresh and dried, once the Introduction Diet has been completed
Shellfish, fresh or frozen
Spices, single and pure without any additives
Spinach
Squash (summer and winter)
Stilton cheese
String beans
Swedes
Swiss cheese
Tangerines

Tea, weak, freshly made, not instant
Tomato puree, pure without any additives apart from salt
Tomato juice, without any additives apart from salt
Tomatoes
Turkey, fresh or frozen
Turnips
Ugly fruit
Uncreamed cottage cheese (dry curd)
Vinegar (cider or white); make sure there is no allergy
Vodka, very occasionally
Walnuts
Watercress
White navy beans, properly prepared
Wine dry: red or white
Yogurt, homemade
Zucchini (courgette)

Dr. Kevin Conners, Dr. Kelly Halderman

What to Expect When You Start DETOXING

Detoxification or cleansing is very misunderstood. Cleansing allows the body to eliminate used wastes and toxins and helps improve our health as it removes harmful substances we inhale, ingest and are exposed to every day.

Most people think of a cleansing program or detox as a way to purge their system of the poor food they have eaten and think of this as a way to lose weight. While it certainly helps with weight loss, cleansing or detoxing is also a valuable and healthy process for those who have undergone heavy pharmaceutical intravenous drugs, or who have been hospitalized. It's also a must for anyone who has (or suspects they have) any food intolerance's and always essential if you've been diagnosed with yeast overgrowth (Candida).

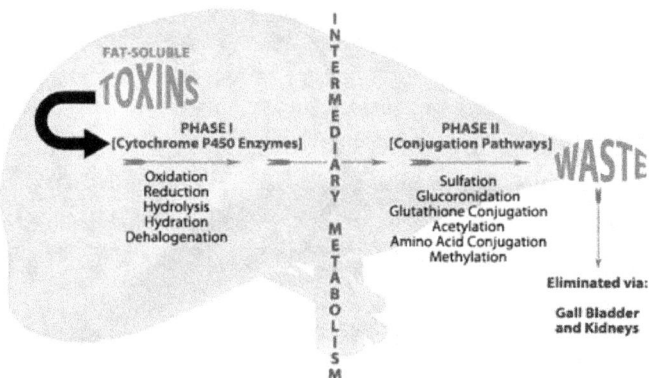

What actually happens when you detox:

Remember that the liver is not only the body's main detoxifying organ it also has a dual role in proper digestion of food. This is why so many people find it very difficult to lose unwanted weight – there livers are overloaded and fat loves to hold on to toxins! When we detoxify our body's liver must convert fat soluble substances to water-soluble (Phase I and Phase II) before they can be eliminated. It's a complicated process to convert these fat soluble toxins to water-soluble ones and involves a number of steps in the metabolic process. Frequently, when people move too quickly, or have problems with some part of this conversion process they end up with toxic metabolites that are far worse than those they were trying to eliminate in the first place. In effect they re-toxify themselves. This is why the Doctor wants you to understand that while SOME symptoms may be expected as NORMAL, having too many is undesirable and you must contact us immediately if this is the case.

What to Expect

Any reaction is an indication that the process of cleansing and detoxification is working and that your body is cleaning itself of impurities, toxins and imbalances.   All reactions are temporary and may occur immediately, within several days or even several weeks later.

But, depending on the levels of toxicity, other possible symptoms are:

- Some people feel ill (flu like complaints) during the first few days of a cleanse because your body is dumping toxins into the blood stream for elimination. The ill-affects usually pass within 1-3 days. On rare occasions, they may last several weeks.

- Sometimes, the discomfort during the healing crisis is of greater intensity than before starting the cleanse.

- Another crisis may come after you begin feeling your very best so remember, health is re-gained in cycles. There may be many small crises to go through before the final outcome is experienced.

- The healing crisis may bring about experiences of past conditions – this is sometimes called RETRACING – going through some of the things that brought you to where you are now. While people often forget the diseases or injuries they have had in the past, they may be reminded during the healing crisis.

- **It is important to note that many people experience little or no discomfort – at all.**

In any case, the cleansing and purifying process is underway, and stored wastes and toxins are in a free-flowing state. The severity and duration of the healing crisis is an indication of amount of toxins and wastes stored in your body. Better out than in! There are a wide variety of reactions (ranging from none to severe) that may manifest during a healing crisis including:

- Increased joint or muscle pain
- Diarrhea
- Constipation
- Fatigue and/or its opposite, restlessness
- Cramps
- Headache
- Aches, Pains
- Insomnia
- Nausea
- Vomiting
- Sinus congestion

- Chills
- Frequent urination and/or urinary tract discharges
- Change in blood pressure
- Skin eruptions, including: boils, hives, and rashes
- Cold or flu-like symptoms
- Strong emotions: anger, despair, sadness, fear
- Suppressed memories
- Anxiety
- Mood swings
- Phobias

Dr. Kevin Conners, Dr. Kelly Halderman
- Fever (usually low grade)

Easing Your Way through the Healing Crisis:
1. Drink plenty of fresh water to flush the body of toxins from the detoxification cleanse. Drink from 1 to 4 quarts (or liters) per day. This will help flush the toxins out of your system and speed along the detoxification.

2. A headache may indicate insufficient water intake … drink more water!

3. Avoid ALL "white" foods: White flour products (bread, pasta, etc.), milk and all dairy products, sugar and starches (white rice, potatoes).

4. Eat MANY lighter meals to keep your blood sugar balanced. Chicken and beef broths, vegetables and soups are especially beneficial.

5. Be kind to yourself, and get the rest that you need. If you are feeling fatigued or sleepy, your body is telling you to rest.

6. On occasion, a reduction of the dosage or temporary cessation may be required until the severity subsides. Call our office.

7. Symptoms frequently disappear immediately after a good bowel movement.

8. COFFEE ENEMAS – 1 – 5 per day!!!!

9. A good massage might be helpful to speed up the healing process and reduce the discomfort.

The benefits of a detoxified, pure body far outweigh any inconveniences that you might experience during the process. Many people describe experiencing *a feeling of lightness*; others are unable to describe what they experience other than to say they can't remember when they felt better.

30 Days on the GAPS Introduction diet

How do I Know When It's Time to Move to The Next Stage on the GAPS Intro?
We recommend moving through intro quickly, and trying new foods and watching for reactions. If necessary due to reactions, go back to the previous stage for a few days/week and then try again. Some individuals dealing with things like seizure disorders, autism, and sever digestion issues may need to stay on some stages longer than others.

Symptoms can be behavioral or physical, watch for anything that went away and then comes back including:

- Diarrhea
- Constipation
- Impulsivity
- Brain Fog
- Tiredness
- Headaches
- Upset Stomach
- Eczema
- Yeast rashes
- Aggressive behavior
- Depression
- Loss of eye contact (and other autism symptoms)
- Stimming (another autism symptom)

Introducing Dairy

Dairy can be introduced during the introduction diet, or not. Introduce dairy products in this order, doing a sensitivity test of placing a drop of the potential food on the wrist of your GAPS patient before bed, allowing it to dry, and then seeing if a reaction occurred overnight.

- Ghee, on the second phase of the intro diet
- Butter, organic and unsalted, after 6 weeks on the diet
- Whey
    - Sensitivity test
    - 1 teaspoon/day of whey added to meat stock or soup
    - After 1-5 days, increase to 2 teaspoons of whey/day
    - Increase whey in this manner until ½ to 1 cup of whey is consumed
- Sour Cream (cultured cream using a yogurt culture)
- Yogurt made with full fat milk
- Kefir and sour cream made with kefir culture

Cheeses allowed on GAPS

Asiago, Brie, Camembert, Cheddar, Colby, Gorgonzola, Gouda, Havarti, Monterey Jack, Muenster, Parmesan, Roquefort, Romano, Stilton, Swiss, Uncreamed cottage cheese (dry curd)

***Start each morning by drinking 1 cup mineral or filtered water and take your PROBIOTIC

Stage 1-

- Meat or fish stock
- Well boiled broccoli, cauliflower, carrots, onions, leeks
- Squash, winter and summer
- Boiled meat

- Sea salt,
- 1-2 teaspoons a day of sauerkraut juice

Stage 2: *Stage 2 allows more foods, but try to introduce them one at a time so that you are sure what you're tolerating and what you're not.*
- Meat or fish stock
- Well boiled GAPS-legal vegetables (no starchy root vegetables)
- Squash, winter and summer
- Boiled meat
- Sea salt
- Fresh herbs
- Fermented vegetables; sauerkraut, kimchi, pickles
- Fermented fish
- Egg yolk, organic, carefully separated from the white
- Homemade ghee
- Stews and casseroles made with meat and vegetables

Stage 3
- Meat or fish stock
- Well boiled GAPS-legal vegetables (no starchy root vegetables)
- Squash, winter and summer
- Boiled meat
- Sea salt
- Fresh herbs
- Fermented vegetables; sauerkraut, kimchi, pickles
- Fermented fish
- Egg yolk, organic, carefully separated from the white
- Homemade ghee
- Stews and casseroles made with meat and vegetables
- Ripe avocado mashed into soups, starting with 1-3 teaspoons a day
- Pancakes made with nutbutter, squash, and eggs- fried in fat or ghee, start with one a day
- Scrambled eggs made with ghee and served with avocado if tolerated and cooked vegetables.

Stage 4
- Meat or fish stock
- Well boiled GAPS-legal vegetables (no starchy root vegetables)
- Squash, winter and summer
- Boiled, roasted, or grilled meat (not burned)
- Sea salt
- Fresh herbs
- Cold pressed olive oil

- Fermented vegetables; sauerkraut, kimchi, pickles
- Fermented fish
- Eggs
- Homemade ghee
- Stews and casseroles made with meat and vegetables
- Ripe avocado
- Pancakes made with nutbutter, squash, and eggs- fried in fat or ghee, start with one a day
- Scrambled eggs made with ghee and served with avocado if tolerated and cooked vegetables.
- Freshly pressed juices, start with a few tablespoons of carrot juice
- Bread made with nut flour, eggs, squash, tolerated fat, salt

Stage 5
- Meat or fish stock
- Raw legal vegetables, peeled
- Squash, winter and summer
- Peeled, cooked apple, pureed
- Honey, up to a couple tablespoons a day
- Boiled, roasted, or grilled meat (not burned)
- Sea salt
- Fresh herbs
- Cold pressed olive oil
- Fermented vegetables; sauerkraut, kimchi, pickles, etc.
- Fermented fish
- Eggs
- Homemade ghee
- Stews and casseroles made with meat and vegetables
- Ripe avocado mashed into soups, starting with 1-3 teaspoons a day
- Pancakes made with nutbutter, squash, and eggs- fried in fat or ghee
- Freshly pressed juices, carrot, mint, cabbage, lettuce, apple, pineapple, mango
- Bread made with nut flour, eggs, squash, tolerated fat, salt

Stage 6
- Meat or fish stock
- Raw legal vegetables, peeled
- Squash, winter and summer
- Peeled, raw apple
- Other fruits, raw, introduce slowly
- Honey, up to a couple tablespoons a day
- Boiled, roasted, or grilled meat (not burned)
- Sea salt

- Fresh herbs
- Cold pressed olive oil
- Fermented vegetables; sauerkraut, kimchi, pickles, etc.
- Fermented fish
- Egg yolk, organic, carefully separated from the white
- Homemade ghee
- Stews and casseroles made with meat and vegetables
- Ripe avocado mashed into soups
- Pancakes made with nutbutter, squash, and eggs- fried in fat or ghee
- Scrambled eggs made with ghee and served with avocado if tolerated and cooked vegetables.
- Freshly pressed juices, carrot, mint, cabbage, lettuce, apple, pineapple, mango
- Bread made with nut flour, eggs, squash, tolerated fat, salt- use dates and dried fruit to sweeten.

Recipes in this guide serve 4 people. Due to the vast differences in the amount people are hungry for on the Intro diet, you may find that you don't need all the food on each day. Within the allowed foods, choices and quantities will be very individual.

Stage 1 Recipes:
Stocks:

Chicken stock:

Ingredients: Whole chicken or chicken pieces

Optional: 2 tablespoons thyme, 6 cloves garlic, 1 onion, 1 inch of ginger root, vegetable scraps such as the ends of onions and carrots, core of the cabbage, leaves from celery, etc

Directions: Rinse chicken. Reach inside cavity and remove giblet package. Remove giblets from package and add to the stock pot. Place chicken in the stockpot. Fill pot ¾ full with filtered water and any optional herbs and vegetables. Cook on medium-high until bubbling, then reduce heat to low and allow to simmer, covered, at least 8 hours. When done, allow to cool then pour stock through a strainer and transfer to mason jars to store in the fridge.

To strain, use a mesh strainer over a pitcher-style 4-cup measuring cup. This makes transferring the stock to the mason jars easier, cleaning out the strainer as needed during the process. Do not discard the soft gelatinous parts around the bones or the skin; reserve that and use an immersion or regular blender to blend it into your stock and soups. The fat will rise to the top of the jars in the fridge, which can be included in soups or used as a fat for cooking. Pick any meat off the bones that you can after the chicken stock has been removed, reserve meat to add to soups or serve alongside. Discard the remaining bones in the pot.

Beef Stock:
Beef marrow bones Filtered water
In a crockpot or stock pot, place 1-2 pounds beef marrow bones and fill to 1 inch from the top with filtered water. Simmer overnight. If there is meat on your stock bones, pull meat off and save for later use.

Lamb Stock:
Ingredients Lamb bones Filtered water
Directions: Fill pot ¾ full with filtered water, add lamb bones. Cook on medium-high until bubbling,

then reduce heat to low and allow to simmer, covered, at least 8 hours. When done, allow to cool then pour stock through a strainer and transfer to mason jars to store in the fridge.

Kimchi
1 Napa cabbage
1 bunch of Green onions 3 Carrots
1 bunch of Radishes
1 tablespoon fresh Ginger, grated 4 cloves of Garlic
4 chili peppers (mild or spicy, depending on your taste preference)
4 teaspoons sea salt
1 teaspoon Whey per mason jar (optional) Makes 4 pint jars full

Aside from the ginger and carrots, which you might want to grate smaller, thinly slice all the vegetables and mix with the salt. Place into jars, pounding down to release juice. Add whey over the top, cover with a lid, and set in a room temperature place to ferment for 2-3 days without opening. Transfer to fridge after that and enjoy now or later.

Sauerkraut
Ingredients:
1 head cabbage, green or purple
2 tablespoons sea salt, course is fine 2 quart sized large-mouth mason jars Food
processor or knife
Cup or cylinder that fits inside the Mason jar, to smash sauerkraut
Directions:
Remove and discard outer leaves of the cabbage, until you get to the clean unblemished leaves underneath. Cut cabbage in half and core. Shred cabbage in food processor using a 'slicing' disk or with a knife, creating thin strips of cabbage. Pack into jars, and add 1 tablespoon salt to each jar. Cover and shake to distribute the salt. Allow to sit out for an hour, until the cabbage wilts. Smash to release juices. Cover again, and allow to ferment on counter for 3 days before transferring to the fridge to store. Sauerkraut is ready to eat after the countertop fermentation.

Veggies:

Intro Butternut Squash Soup
2 quarts stock
1 quart filtered water
4 cups pre-cut butternut squash cubes 1 tablespoon sea salt (adjust to taste)

Simmer all ingredients to make a soup. Puree with an immersion blender if desired for a smooth soup

Boiled Broccoli
Simmer 2-4 cups of broccoli until soft. Sprinkle with sea salt, top with the fat that rose to the top of your chicken stock.

Onion Leek Soup
1 quarts stock
1 quart water
5 onions, sliced
4 leeks, sliced
2 cloves garlic, crushed
1 tablespoon sea salt (or to taste)

Simmer everything for one hour or overnight on low in the crockpot.

Squash chunks
4 cups squash chunks

Dr. Kevin Conners, Dr. Kelly Halderman

4 tablespoons animal fat (lamb, beef, chicken, etc) Sprinkle of sea salt

In a saucepan with a lid, simmer squash in enough water to cover for 30 minutes, or until very soft. Drain gently and top with fat and salt.

Sweet Onions
6-8 small onions
1 quart stock
1 teaspoon sea salt

Simmer small peeled whole onions in enough stock to cover for one hour, covered, until soft all the way through. Reserve leftover stock for soup.
Creamy Cauliflower
2 pounds cauliflower
1 quart stock
½ teaspoon salt
4 tablespoons lamb tallow

Boil cauliflower until soft, 20 minutes. Drain, reserving stock for use in soup. "Butter" the cauliflower with tallow and sprinkle with salt.

Boiled Squash
Boil bite sized squash pieces until soft. Top with tallow and salt.

Summer Squash Soup
2 quarts stock
1 quart filtered water
8 small summer squash; crookneck, zucchini, patty pan, etc.
1 tablespoon sea salt (adjust to taste)

Remove stems and blossom ends from squash, coarsely chop. Simmer all ingredients to make a soup. Puree with an immersion blender if desired for a smooth soup.

Meats:

Chicken meat with Soup
Gently heat chicken left from stock in a steamer or by boiling in water. Top with Butternut squash soup, or dip in the soup.

Boiled Steak:
Boil 6-8 steaks, sprinkle with salt.

Meat Patties
3 pounds hamburger
3 carrots and 1 cup cauliflower, shredded 2 cups stock
½ teaspoon sea salt

Form hamburger into patties; simmer in stock with the vegetables until cooked through. Blend the veggies into the stock after removing the patties, and serve as a 'sauce' over the top.

Meat Strips
1 roast, 4 pounds
2 quarts water
2 teaspoon sea salt

Slice roast into 'jerky' like strips, and simmer meat strips in water with salt for 30 minutes or until cooked

Dr. Kevin Conners, Dr. Kelly Halderman

through.

Beef and Broccoli Soup
1 quarts beef stock
1-2 cups fish stock (*optional*) 1 quart filtered water
1 tablespoon sea salt (to taste)
2 cloves garlic, peeled and crushed 2 pounds broccoli
2 pounds beef roast, or meat from stock bones if your bones came with meat like mine do.

In a crockpot or in a stockpot combine stock, water, salt, garlic, and broccoli. Simmer 1 hour Or until broccoli is very soft. Blend with an immersion blender until smooth. Add back in beef and heat until warm, or chop a beef roast into bite sized pieces and simmer until cooked through.

Boiled Meatballs with carrots and onions
3 pounds ground meat 1 carrot
1 onion
½ teaspoon sea salt

Puree or grate carrot and onion, mix with meat and salt and form into balls. Simmer in stock or water. Reserve water or stock from simmering to add for soup.

Stage 2 Recipes:

Introduce: Start with 1 teaspoon fermented vegetable; kimchi or sauerkraut.

Homemade ghee
1 pound unsalted butter, or more as desired
Preheat oven to 140-250* Place butter in an oven proof dish or pan. Bake for 45-60 minutes, take out very carefully, and pour the golden fat from the top, being careful to leave the white milk solids in the pan. Keep in a glass jar and refrigerate. You can save the buttery milk solids for others who eat butter in the house, or discard.

Crispy Walnuts:
To soak nuts: Place 2-3 lbs raw nuts in a large bowl (they will swell, so only fill 2/3 full, using another bowl if needed). Add 2 tablespoons sea salt and cover the nuts with filtered water. Allow to soak overnight at room temperature (on the counter). No need to cover. To dry: Drain in a colander and start dehydrating the nuts you soaked last night, or roast in a pan as low as your oven will go. Dehydrate all day.

Zucchini casserole
1 pounds chicken, cubed 4 zucchinis
1 teaspoon sea salt
½ cup stock

Cube chicken in bite sized pieces. Slice zucchini into
¼ inch rounds. Place chicken and stock in the bottom of a loaf pan, sprinkle with salt, and top with zucchini rounds. Cover with foil and bake at 350* for 45 minutes, or until chicken is cooked through and zucchini is soft.

Butternut Squash and Beef Casserole
1 pounds hamburger
1 large butternut squash (3 pounds)
½ teaspoon sea salt 2 cups stock
Tallow or fat to grease pan

Dr. Kevin Conners, Dr. Kelly Halderman

Preheat oven to 350* Mix hamburger with sea salt. Peel and remove pulp from butternut squash, and chop into bite-sized pieces. Grease a 9x13" pan with fat. Place squash in the pan and pour stock over the squash. Place pieces of the raw hamburger over the top of the squash, covering evenly. Bake uncovered for 45 minutes or until squash is soft and beef is cooked.

Boiled Meatballs with Garlic and Parsley
3 pounds hamburger
3 carrots and 1 cup cauliflower, shredded 3 cloves garlic, minced or crushed
3 sprigs fresh parsley, finely chopped 2 cups stock
½ teaspoon sea salt

Mix hamburger with vegetables, garlic, and parsley. Simmer in stock with added sea salt, gently turning as needed, until cooked through.

Stuffed Peppers
6 bell peppers
1-2 pounds assorted vegetables (carrot, onion, broccoli, cauliflower), shredded
3 pounds ground meat, raw
½ teaspoon sea salt

Mix veggies, meat, and salt. Wash and cut tops off bell peppers, rinse out seeds. Stuff meat evenly into bell peppers. Place in a casserole dish with a lid, add ½ inch water to the bottom. Bake at 350* for one hour covered, or until meat is cooked through and peppers are soft. Serve.

Egg Drop Soup
6 leeks, sliced
1 quart fish stock
1 quart other stock 2 teaspoons sea salt 4 onions, sliced
4 egg yolks, beaten with a fork

Wash and slice the leeks up to where the leaves separate (use the light parts) and peel and slice the onions thinly. Simmer in stock with salt until soft, 1 hour. Raise heat to a rapid boil and gently drip in a thin stream of egg yolks, whisking with a fork as you pour them in to make 'noodles'. Remove from heat and serve.

Chunky Chicken Soup
1 pound carrots
1 winter or summer squash, peeled, and cut into cubes
Cooked chicken, cubed 1 quart stock
1 quart filtered water 1 teaspoon sea salt

Simmer chopped veggies in stock and water until soft. Add chicken and heat until warm.

Slow Cooked Pulled Brisket
4 onions or equivalent of other veggies, peeled and sliced
Brisket roast, 3-4 pounds 1 cup stock
½ teaspoon sea salt
In a slow cooker, place sliced onions. Put brisket roast on top and pour stock over. Sprinkle sea salt over roast. Cook on low all day or on high for 4 hours. Remove brisket and puree the onions and stock/drippings into 'gravy' and then place the brisket back in and pull apart with two forks, mixing the gravy in.

Dr. Kevin Conners, Dr. Kelly Halderman

Stage 3 Recipes:

Ginger Tea
1 inch ginger root, peeled and sliced into thin coins 2 quarts filtered water

Simmer ginger root in water for 10 minutes, covered. Enjoy warm or cool and enjoy cold.

Summer Squash Intro Pancakes (can add 1 cup of crispy nuts to recipe)
   1 small crookneck squash 2 eggs
1 teaspoon tallow to fry in

In a blender, blend squash and eggs until smooth. Heat a skillet on medium-low heat and melt lamb tallow. Make small pancakes with the batter, and carefully flip once set on one side, after 90 seconds or so.

Butternut Squash Pancakes
   1 small butternut squash or other winter squash 2 cups crispy walnuts
6 eggs
   1 teaspoon tallow to fry in

Peel and chop raw squash, or use cooked. In a blender, blend squash, walnuts, and eggs until smooth. Heat a skillet on medium-low heat and melt tallow. Make small pancakes with the batter, and carefully flip once set on one side, after 90 seconds or so.

Boiled Green Beans
1 pound green beans, simmered 2 cloves garlic, crushed
4 tablespoons tallow

Taco Salad Casserole
   4 tomatoes
2 pounds Steak (sirloin tip is good) 2 onions
½ teaspoon sea salt
 1 Anaheim chili, diced 1 cup stock

In a casserole dish, layer slices of tomatoes, cubes of steak, slices of onion. Sprinkle with chili and sea salt. Pour stock over. Cover and bake at 350* for 45 minutes. Top with

Fresh cilantro
 2 cloves garlic, crushed 1 avocado, pureed
And serve.

Intro Broccoli Beef Soup
   4 pounds hamburger
2 pounds broccoli
2 pounds cauliflower
2 quarts stock
1 tablespoon sea salt

Simmer all ingredients, breaking up hamburger as it cooks.

Simmered Burgers
 1 pounds ground beef
½ teaspoon sea salt
½ teaspoon pepper 2 cups stock

Dr. Kevin Conners, Dr. Kelly Halderman

Mix seasonings into beef and form into patties. Simmer in stock and top with guacamole.

Guacamole:
Ingredients:
2-3 ripe avocados
2 cloves garlic
1/2 teaspoon sea salt

Directions:
Press two cloves of garlic through a garlic press. Add in 1 teaspoon of cumin, ½ a teaspoon of salt, the juice of one lemon, mix. Mash in 2-3 ripe avocados with a fork. If storing, press plastic wrap right up against the guacamole to help prevent it from oxidizing and turning brown, store in the fridge for a couple hours

Stage 4 Recipes:

Freshly Pressed Carrot Juice
Juice 1-2 carrots and try 2-3 tablespoons of carrot juice, can be mixed in with water or consumed on its own.

Scrambled Eggs with Vegetables
10 eggs, whisked
2 tablespoons tallow or ghee
¼ teaspoon sea salt 2 onions, sliced
2 avocado

In a skillet, melt tallow over medium heat. Sautee onions until soft, approx. 20 minutes. Add salt and eggs, and scramble eggs until nearly cooked through, remove before they are cooked all the way through to prevent from turning dry. Top with chunks of avocado or pureed avocado.

Intro Breakfast Sausage
 3 lbs ground beef
2 cloves garlic, crushed
¼ inch ginger, grated or diced
Combination of fresh basil, parsley, cilantro, or other fresh herbs, finely chopped, 2-6 tablespoons 1 teaspoons sea salt

Combine beef with seasonings, form into patties, and fry in a pan or simmer in stock until cooked through.

Intro Nut Flour Bread
 1 cups almond flour 6 eggs
2 cups butternut squash, peeled (the neck of one medium squash)
1 teaspoon sea salt
6 tablespoons tallow to grease muffin pan

Puree all ingredients in a blender or food processor (you can keep the zucchini raw and just puree). Pour into greased muffin tins or a small loaf pan. Bake at 350* for 20 minutes, or until a knife inserted comes out clean.

Chili Chicken
4 pounds chicken thighs
2 Anaheim chilies, deseeded 2 cloves garlic
 1 tablespoon fresh parsley, chopped

½ teaspoon sea salt 1 quart stock

Rinse chicken and place in the bottom of a lidded casserole dish. Pour stock over the chicken, top chicken with finely diced chili, crushed garlic, parsley and sea salt. Cover and cook at 350* for 1 hour or until cooked through.

Olive Oil and Fresh Herb Blend
1 quart cold pressed olive oil 1 bunch (4 ounces) basil
½ teaspoon sea salt
1-10 cloves garlic (optional)

In a blender place basil, salt, garlic, and as much olive oil as can fit. Puree until smooth. Use this 'pesto sauce' as a tasty way to get cold pressed olive oil into your meals.

Stuffed Tomatoes
2 pounds ground beef
1 pound beef or chicken liver
2 cloves garlic, crushed
½ teaspoon sea salt
Fresh herbs as desired, 1 tablespoon (basil, parsley, etc)
6 large tomatoes

In a food processor, pulse to chop liver. Add to ground beef and mix in seasonings. Cut the tops off the tomatoes, and scoop out membranes and seeds using a spoon. Fill with beef mixture. Bake in a casserole dish, uncovered, for 30 minutes or until meat is cooked through. Drizzle with herbed olive oil and serve.

Veggie Stew
2 quarts chicken stock
2 pounds cubed stew meat
4 leeks, washed and sliced, just the white and light green parts
4 summer squash, chopped 2 onions, sliced
1 tablespoon sea salt (to taste) 2 carrots, cut into matchsticks 1 cup snow peas

Directions: Heat a soup pot or skillet to medium high heat, sprinkle meat with salt, then brown all sides of the meat, stirring, for about 10 minutes. Add stock, leeks, summer squash, onions, carrots, and salt and simmer for 1-2 hours. Add in snow peas 20 minutes before serving.

Salmon Patties
2 pounds wild caught salmon, fresh or frozen 1 egg
½ teaspoon sea salt
Tallow or ghee to fry

In a pan with a lid, cook salmon over medium heat, turning once, until cooked through. Once salmon is cooked, allow to cool briefly (you can also just eat the salmon as is if you'd like) and then flake it with a fork, mix in the egg and salt, and form into patties. Fry over medium heat in tallow or ghee until a golden brown, approx. 5 minutes on each side.

Stage 5 Recipes:

Apple Sauce
6 ripe apples
½ cup filtered water

Peel and core apples. Thinly slice and simmer in a saucepan with the water, covered, until very soft. Mash with a fork and eat with ghee or tallow.

Dr. Kevin Conners, Dr. Kelly Halderman

Egg and Squash Bake
6 eggs
1 neck of a medium butternut squash 1 teaspoon sea salt
1 tablespoon tallow

Peel squash and cut into chunks. Puree or grate in food processor. Add in eggs and sea salt. Grease 8x8 glass dish with tallow and pour in egg mixture. Bake at 350* for 20 minutes, or until set in the center.

Butter Lettuce Salad
1 head butter lettuce, torn 1 tomato, cubed
1 onion, diced

Mix salad and top with bacon if desired and dressing below.

Basil Garlic Dressing
This is similar to the herbed olive oil and can be poured over foods as well

4 ounces fresh basil
3 cups cold pressed olive oil
6 cloves garlic

Puree all ingredients, using a quart small mouth mason jar fitted with the blender blade if desired. Pour over salads and meats.

Roast Vegetables
1 pound cauliflower florets 3 large carrots
1 celery root, peeled and chopped (optional) 3 stalks of celery, chopped
 1 pound asparagus, chopped (if in season)
¼ cup olive oil
½ teaspoon sea salt
 2 tablespoons dried basil or other seasoning blend

Toss veggies with sea salt, olive oil, and seasoning. Place into a 9x13 " glass oven safe dish. Cook at 400 Degrees for 45 minutes

Drumsticks
8 Chicken drumsticks
6 summer squash
4 onions, peeled and quartered Sea salt to taste

Bake drumsticks (or roast a whole chicken) surrounded by chopped squash and onions for 30 minutes, or until cooked through. Reserve bones for stock.

Meatballs
These meatballs are packed with veggies for flavor, moisture, and nutrition
3 pounds ground beef (or other ground meat) 1 carrot
1 onion
1 zucchini
 1 teaspoon sea salt
½ teaspoons freshly ground black pepper
¼ cup onion gravy from yesterday

Using a food processor or grater, grate the carrot, onion, and zucchini. Mix in with the meat, adding in salt and pepper. Form into balls. Pour gravy over meatballs and then bake at 375* for 30 minutes, or until cooked through.

Grilled Crispy Bacon

Dr. Kevin Conners, Dr. Kelly Halderman

1 pound bacon, sugar and nitrate free (we use beef bacon from US Wellness)

On a large griddle over two burners, or in two skillets, fry bacon over medium heat. Turn once the edges start to brown. Once cooked, remove to paper towels to drain, serve warm.
Reserve bacon drippings in the fridge to use for cooking later on- bacon drippings add a fantastic flavor to just about anything!

Stock and Onion Gravy
1 pot chicken stock
6 onions, peeled and sliced 1 teaspoon sea salt

Simmer onions in chicken stock, covered, until onions are soft. Add 1 teaspoon sea salt and puree with an immersion blender. Remove lid and reduce over low heat until desired consistency (reduced by half is good). Store in glass jars in the fridge and spoon over meats, add to scrambled eggs, and use to sauté veggies in.

Baked Salmon
 2 wild-caught salmon filets - about a pound each 2 Tablespoons Dill
2 Tablespoons Thyme 1/2 teaspoon pepper 1/2 teaspoon sea salt
1 teaspoon olive oil

Directions:
Heat the oven to 200 F. (not a typo) Mix dill, thyme, pepper, and sea salt.

Beef Roast in the Crockpot

1 beef roast, 3-6 lbs
1 pound pearl onions, peeled 4 carrots, cut into chunks
6 summer squash, cut into chunks 4 cloves garlic, crushed
1 sprig fresh rosemary 1 tablespoon sea salt

In a crock pot, place beef roast. Cover with garlic and rosemary. Place vegetables around beef, and sprinkle everything with sea salt. Cook on low all day or high for 4 hours. Spoon drippings over beef to serve.

Stage 6 Recipes:

Freshly Pressed Juice
Juice:
1 bunch celery
 1 bunch parsley
 2 carrots
2 green apples

Fruit Salad
4 apples
4 pears
4 ripe bananas

Apple Chutney
Apples, peeled and chopped; to fill a quart jar (6 or so)
Juice of 2 lemons
2 tablespoons honey 1/2 cup raisins
 2 inches of hot chili pepper, fresh and de-seeded 1 teaspoon fennel seeds

Dr. Kevin Conners, Dr. Kelly Halderman

Mix all ingredients, place in jar. Pack gently to start to release the juices. If needed, add filtered water to cover the fruit. Cover and leave at room temperature for 2 days, transferring to the refrigerator for up to 2 months.
Discard the chili pepper after the 2-day fermentation at room temperature.

Raw Apple and Cabbage Salad

1 apple, peeled and shredded
¼ cabbage head, shredded
½ teaspoon fresh ginger, peeled and diced Toss ingredients together.

Zucchini Bread
2 cups almond flour 6 eggs
2-3 medium zucchini
½ teaspoon sea salt 2 tablespoons tallow

Puree all ingredients in a blender or food processor (you can keep the zucchini raw and just puree).
Pour into greased muffin tins or a small loaf pan. Bake at 350* for 30-45 minutes, or until a knife inserted comes out clean.

'Meal' Salad
Meal salads are wonderful for spring and summer. Crunchy greens with lots of toppings.

1 pound greens; spinach, lettuce, cabbage 2 tomatoes, chopped
1 onion, diced
1 cup crispy nuts, chopped
½ cup sunflower seeds
1 pound chicken, cooked, sliced

Layer all ingredients and toss with dressing right before serving. Top with herbed olive oil.

Butternut Squash and Beef Casserole

1 pounds hamburger
1 large butternut squash (3 pounds)
½ teaspoon sea salt 2 cups stock
Tallow or fat to grease pan

Preheat oven to 350* Mix hamburger with sea salt. Peel and remove pulp from butternut squash, and chop into bite-sized pieces. Grease a 9x13" pan with fat. Place squash in the pan and pour stock over the squash. Place pieces of the raw hamburger over the top of the squash, covering evenly. Bake uncovered for 45 minutes or until squash is soft and beef is cooked.

Chicken Curry Soup
1 tablespoons tallow or ghee 1 Anaheim chili
4 onions, sliced
½ inch ginger root, peeled and grated 1 quart stock
1 quart filtered water
4 cups cooked chicken, diced 6 cloves garlic, crushed

In the bottom of a pot, sauté onions, ginger, and pepper in tallow until onions are soft. Add stock and water and bring to a simmer. Add chicken and cook 20 minutes, or until heated through. Top with garlic and serve.

Dr. Kevin Conners, Dr. Kelly Halderman

Meatball-vegetable soup:
Ingredients:
1 quart chicken stock, 4 teaspoons sea salt, 1 quart filtered water, 8-10 meatballs,
4 cups of chopped vegetables (broccoli, carrots, onions, spinach, tomatoes, squash; whatever combination you'd like).

Directions:
Add stock, water, salt, tomato paste, vegetables to crock pot and cook on low all day. Add meatballs during the last 30 minutes of cooking to heat thoroughly. When serving, evenly distribute meatballs among bowls with the soup.

Baked Honey Mustard Chicken

2 pounds boneless chicken thighs
¼ cup prepared mustard, natural 2 tablespoons honey
2 tablespoons tallow

Grease a 9x13 glass casserole with tallow. Preheat oven to 375*. Mix mustard and honey in a shallow dish and coat chicken with it. Place chicken in casserole dish, skin side up if there is skin, and bake for 35 minutes or until juices run clear.

More on Barrier Breakdown and Healing

For the Doctor

Local Inflammation – is increased in vessels and kidneys as demonstrated with lab values showing increased hsCRP (IL-1b, IL-6, TNFalpha), leucocytosis, increased Neutrophils, and increased Lymphocytes. Increased RAAS (renin-angiotensin-aldosterone system) reveals inflammation in the Kidneys commonly due to endothelial damage. It is helpful to measure these markers.

Oxidative Stress (ROS (Radical Oxygen Species) and RNS (Radical Nitrogen Species)) is increased in arteries and kidneys along with a decreased oxidative defense. Autoimmune dysfunction of the arteries and kidneys will reveal increased WBCs, involvement of CD4+ and CD8+, Th1/Th2 dominance as measured by cytokines and elevated CRP.

As stated, the intimal lining is a continuous parallel sheet of cells, an interface between the blood vessel and blood (lumen). It releases vasoactive substances that regulate all endothelial function, vascular smooth muscle (VSM), and affecting the circulating blood.

Its major function is to maintain appropriate vasomotor tone, especially in the coronary arteries and systemic resistance arteries. It is a living barrier maintaining vascular homeostasis allowing selective permeability, acting as a monitor and transducer of blood-borne signals, is a source and target of physiological response modifiers, an integrator of local pathophysiologic milieu, and offers dynamic regulation of hemostasis and thrombosis, vascular growth and remodeling, and inflammatory and immune reactions. So, please don't tell me it's not important in brain-based patients! For the sake of this discussion, we will keep content associated to the intima's role in inflammation and autoimmune control.

Endothelial receptors are transmembrane proteins on the cell membrane that specifically or selectively bind to extracellular (intraluminal) ligands. Several types of receptors have been identified as frequent participants in signaling endothelial hyper-permeability, including receptor tyrosine kinases (RTKs), G-protein-coupled receptors (GPCRs), and integrin receptors. An example of RTKs would be the receptors of many growth factors, e.g., fibroblast growth factor (FGF) and VEGF. VEGF (vascular endothelial growth factor) is an angiogenic cytokine (increases growth of new vessels) that was initially identified as a potent endothelial permeability-increasing factor. VEGF-induced hyper-permeability is involved in tumor development, diabetic retinopathy, and ischemia/reperfusion injury. VEGF binds to tyrosine kinase receptor subtypes. Practically speaking, healing the BBB would involve down-regulating VEGF-RTKs.

> *"To survive and prosper, we must think differently and make different choices than we have made in the past."*
> - *Margaret M. Polski, Wired for Survival*

Many permeability-increasing agents (e.g., histamine, thrombin, or bradykinin) signal through GPCRs. Each type of GPCR is coupled to a specific subtype of G-protein, which will initiate specific series of intracellular signaling events. Thrombin is a serine protease that cleaves fibrinogen into fibrin forming the base for blood clots during intrinsic or extrinsic (caused by injury) activation of coagulation. Thrombin also induces endothelial hyper-permeability by binding to protease-activated receptors (PARs) on the endothelial cell surface.

Bradykinin is produced during inflammation or ischemia/reperfusion injury. Occupancy of the bradykinin B2 receptor on microvascular endothelial cells increases cytosolic $Ca2+$ via similar mechanisms to those of the histamine H1 receptor or PAR-1, and activates membrane-bound phospholipase A2 (PLA2) to produce arachidonic acid (AA). AA metabolism by lipoxygenase and cyclooxygenase (COX) produces leukotrienes, prostanglandins, and thromboxin A2. Most of these metabolites have been shown to cause endothelial dysfunction.

Peroxidative mechanisms have consistently been implicated in demyelinating diseases, and the application of antioxidants has been shown to offer clinical improvements. Though the majority of investigations into the role of these redox imbalances have focused on direct damage to the myelin (in MS and ALS patients) the initial oxidative stress is happening at the vascular level, then the astrocyte border, followed by direct attack on oligodendricytes. Increased BBB permeability does result from increased free radicals entering the CNS, so the subsequent administration of antioxidants can restore balance at all three levels.

Sources of oxidative stress need to be identified and addressed as the initial cause is usually distant from the BBB. An often overlooked source of oxidative stress is imbalanced hepatic detoxification, wherein Phase I detoxification exceeds the capacity of Phase II detoxification and a buildup of exudate follows. As a result, numerous free radicals are generated. Think of things like Alpha-lipoic acid (ALA), N-Acetyl L Cysteine, Cordyceps, Gotu Kola, Fish Oils (I suggest a balanced mix), Quercetin, Stinging Nettle, Rutin, Bromelain, and Curcumin.

Intracellular messenger cAMP improves endothelial barrier function and protects microvasculature from hyper-permeability. Nitric oxide (NO) is a short-lived free radical produced in response to phosphorylation and activation of nitric oxide synthase (NOS). Three isoforms of NOS have been implicated in inflammatory responses: endothelial (eNOS; NOS1), inducible (iNOS; NOS2), and neuronal (nNOS; NOS3). The role of NO in regulating endothelial barrier function is controversial. NO has opposing effects on endothelial permeability depending upon the endothelial tissue examined but is thought to have a role of vasodilation in in both the heart and the brain. NO serves as a vasodilator and factors that stimulate NO production should be considered. Think of using natural Calcium and Sodium channel blockers such as Hawthorn, Cornflower, Centaury, Lemon Balm, Motherwort, and Valerian Root. Garlic, Calcium, Magnesium, CoQ10, Fish oils, L-arginine, and L-citrulline are also things to consider.

In order to help Nitric Oxide to work properly, co-factors essential for function include Calmodulin, BH4 – tetrahydrobiopterin, Flavin Redox co-factors (FAD, FMN),Glutatione precursors, ALA, NAC, Whey protein, Niacinamide, Thiol and Sulfydryal groups, SNO (S-nitrosothiols) – organosulfur coumpounds also known as Mercaptans as they bond so strongly to Hg (Garlic, MSM, and ALA).

Metal-NO Complexes are very mineral dependent so Zinc and Copper deficiencies can offset gain in stimulating production. Also, because of the NO-metal complex, heavy metal toxicity can displace minerals and lead to greater damage in NO function. Clinical pearl – heavy metal toxicity interrupts NO function as the heavy metals displace Zinc and Copper in the metal-NO complex. Unfortunately, people take elemental Iron for anemia and Iodine for thyroid issues that also bind to NO complexes and cause problems. Only use plant-source minerals!!! People's Centrum can actually be causing their BBB disruption and their high blood pressure!

Protein phosphorylation regulated by protein kinases and phosphatases is a major determinant of endothelial barrier function. However, kinase-dependent signaling can be exceptionally complex being that there are more than 500 protein kinases in the human genome.

Inflammatory eicosanoids, such as prostaglandin E2 (PGE2) derived from arachidonic acid, may also be responsible for disrupting the BBB. Research shows a significantly higher production of PGE2 in patients with chronic progressive brain-based disorders. Lab lipid profiles of these patients reveal staggering deficiencies of omega-3 fatty acids, precursors of the less inflammatory PGE3. It makes one think that dietary changes in fatty acid intake to modulate prostaglandin production remain essential to integrative treatment protocols. Also, natural agents that block the actions of cyclooxygenase (COX) and 5-lipoxygenase can help prevent BBB disruptions; however, using pharmaceuticals like that block COX2 with ramp-up PGE2 and cause more distruction. This is the scuttlebutt about . Nutritional considerations that block these enzymes include bromelain, pancreatic enzyme, curcumin, ginger, quercetin, and other bioflavonoids.

Matrix metalloproteinases are a family of 29 proteases that are dependent upon metal (zinc) ions for their proteolytic activity. Activated MMPs cleave components of the endothelial extracellular matrix during normal remodeling and maintenance of the basement membrane and can cause microvascular barrier dysfunction under pathophysiological conditions like local infiltration of antigens or cytokines from a distant inflammatory process. Here is another example of cell barrier damage downstream from a primary immune stimulation event.

> *Your time is limited, so don't waste it living someone else's life. Don't be trapped by dogma - which is living with the results of other people's thinking. Don't let the noise of others' opinions drown out your own inner voice. And most important, have the courage to follow your heart and intuition.*
>
> Steve Jobs

ADAMs (a disintegrin and metalloproteinases) are a family of 40 known genes, encoding at least 21 human functional proteins involved in tumor metastasis, angiogenesis, and inflammation. During inflammation, ADAM15 mediates endothelial hyper-permeability via a mechanism that does not require the proteolytic activity of its extracellular domain [435]. Rather, the cytosolic C-terminus initiates signaling through Src kinase and ERK1/2 to signal endothelial hyperpermeability. This signaling mechanism contributes to microvascular fluid leakage in the lungs of mice in response to systemic exposure to bacterial endotoxin (lipopolysaccharide), and is involved in pneumonia-induced lung injury in humans

Matrix metalloproteinases (MMPs) are enzymes, secreted by immune cells, which can dissolve components of the extracellular matrix. For most parts of the body, these actions are useful in allowing white blood cells access to areas of injury or infection. However, release of these enzymes in CNS capillaries can result in BBB breakdown. Inhibition of these enzymes should be considered.

Flavonoids, well-known for their capillary-strengthening effects, can inhibit the activity of MMPs. Flavonoids, particularly proanthocyanidins and anthocyanins, are taken up into the cellular matrix. Receptor sites on the flavonoids bind metalloproteinase enzymes, thereby preventing their liquefying effect on the matrix. Bilberry anthocyanosides have been shown to restore damaged BBB permeability. Flavonoids are also highly anti-inflammatory and potent antioxidants, giving you another reason to eat your fruits and vegetables. Supplementation consideration should include bilberry (with 25% anthocyanin content, 80-160 mg. tid). Grape seed or pine bark extracts (150-300 mg/day) can be added for their proanthocyandin content, Bugleweed, Calendula, and Green Tea extract.

Understand that etiological theories of brain disorders, let's use MS as an example, concentrate on a systemic immune response damaging intra-CNS structures. Research has shown that the development of myelin-sensitized lymphocytes as a causative factor but if the patient had an intact BBB, this would be irrelevant, because normally the blood-brain barrier (BBB) denies these cells access to the brain and spinal cord. This brings us back to a dysfunction of the BBB contributes to MS.

Also understand that the vascular barrier that first must be penetrated undergoes moment-to-moment changes at the cytoskeleton, cell–cell junction complexes, and cell attachments to extracellular matrix and basement membrane. Appropriate regulation of these events maintains a low and selective permeability to fluid and solutes under normal physiological conditions. As we discussed, endothelial barrier dysfunction occurs during stimulation by inflammatory agents, pathogens, activated blood cells, endogenous cytokines, heavy metal or other toxins (vaccinations), or other disease states.

This explains why two individuals given the same dose of toxin would/could react very different as far as the effect on the CNS. If the blood-brain barrier is not working properly to screen out and prevent entry of unwanted immunological agents/toxins into the CNS, that individual will experience greater influx of toxic substances in the brain. Hence, a person with myelin-sensitized lymphocytes, who also experiences a weakening of the BBB, is likely to develop MS symptoms with the severity of symptoms depending on the extent of BBB disruption. Individuals with a rapid, "galloping" progression of MS may actually be displaying a pronounced BBB dysfunction. In contrast, those who have a slow, relapsing/remitting course may have periods of better BBB integrity. Carry this same example to any brain based disorder.

Thiamin is known to strengthen the blood-brain barrier, and thiamin deficiencies have been demonstrated to result in problems. Who in the world would have a thiamin deficiency today? Well, it's worse than you'd think. Supplementation of synthetic B vitamins as are used in nearly every OTC B supplement as were as added B vitamins in foods that are 'fortified' is exactly what can cause a B vitamin deficiency! Counter-think? Well, though synthetic B vitamins (made from coal tar derivatives) may act similar to natural B vitamins in some people, in many they do not. BBB compromise due to hypothiaminosis is manifested by loosening cell-to-cell adhesion of vascular endothelial cells and allowing immunoglobulins to pass across the BBB. Every brain-base patient should consider a natural source B vitamin – we use Premiere Research Labs and

Dr. Kevin Conners, Dr. Kelly Halderman

Standard Process Labs. These give the patient the added benefit in supporting liver detoxification pathways as well.

Elevated blood homocysteine levels are known for their association with cardiovascular disease, but homocysteine is equally a vascular toxin in cerebrovascular damage. As with thiamin deficiency, the B vitamins along with folate in the form of 5-methyltetrahydrafolate are key homocysteine-reducing nutrients.

Platelet activating factor (PAF), and inflammatory cytokine, is produced by endothelial cells (also by platelets, monocytes, and macrophages). PAF increases BBB permeability. Some natural agents to consider that have been shown to inhibit PAF include decosahexanoic acid (DHA) from fish oil, and Ginkgo biloba which are potent PAF antagonists. One experimental study of 10 patients with MS in acute relapse who received therapy with Ginkgo (80mg, tid) led to improved neurological scores in 80% of patients.

Summary for Patients

Our understanding of the anatomy and physiology of the BBB is still in its infancy. There is much to learn about the role of the BBB in the pathogenesis of MS. Certainly, it still makes sense to focus on the modulation of the immune aspects of the disease. However, addressing the dynamics of BBB integrity may improve the efficacy of treatments for MS. Complementary therapies that protect BBB integrity may provide an excellent adjunct to conventional therapies.

Natural supplements to consider to help heal BBB permeability:

- Whole-food Vitamin B (we use Premiere Research Labs and Stand Process – these have the proper type of folate in them)
- Phosphatidylserine (PS)
- Ginkgo
- Alpha Lipoic Acid (ALA)
- Whole-food Vitamin C
- Vitamin E (gamma tocopherol and the tocotrienols)
- Bilberry
- Grape seed extract
- Pine bark extract
- Pycnogenol
- Bromelain
- Curcumin

Dr. Kevin Conners, Dr. Kelly Halderman

- o Ginger
- o Quercetin
- o Omega 3 Fish Oils
- o Bugleweed
- o Calendula
- o Pancreatic enzymes
- o N-Acetyl L Cysteine
- o Cordyceps and other medicinal mushrooms
- o Stinging Nettle
- o Rutin
- o Whey protein
- o Niacinamide
- o Thiol and Sulfydryal groups
- o Garlic
- o MSM
- o Minerals – especially Zinc and Copper

There are different products on the market that contain a variety of the above ingredients aimed at healing the damaged borders. It has always been our opinion to seek appropriate medical care from a qualified functional medical doctor/neurologist before embarking on any protocol and, once again, this book is meant to lay out a general understanding and not meant to be a protocol to follow without the help of a physician.

If you need help finding a qualified physician, please e-mail us at the email listed below. We see patients from around the world that fly in to Minnesota and spend a week or so with us but we also understand that we cannot possibly see everyone in need. This is why we've taught doctor seminars and have added a link on our website for practitioner education.

Again, seek more information on our website where you can download ALL of Dr. Conners books and much more helpful data:

www.UpperRoomWellness.com

upperroomwc@gmail.com

B) Finding and Fixing the SOURCE

For the Doctor

Chronic Gram-Negative Bacterial Infections

The effects of chronic inflammatory cytokines in tissues due to gram-negative bacteria are grossly destructive and seldom addressed as cause. Depending on the tissue involved, patients will be properly diagnosed with a disease that improperly omits the source. Biomarkers that hint at gram-negative bacterial infiltration are elevated CRP, elevated Homocysteine, elevated inflammatory cytokines, elevated white cells, and other inflammatory markers but none are specifically definitive and the doctor must discern from the overall picture of the patient.

For example, elevated C-reactive protein (CRP), homocysteine and inflammatory cytokines such as interleukin-6 (IL-6) are associated with increased cardiovascular risk as homocysteine increases the production of MCP-1 and IL-8 in endothelial cells. These are just signs however, like a crossed, double-R warning of a railroad crossing. Most doctors will warn their patients of the cardiovascular risk, administer treatment for associated signs such as high blood pressure or abnormal lipids and completely ignore the roaring train ready to crush the patient's vehicle sitting on the tracks.

In the CNS, chronic microglial activation contributes to neuronal damage in neurodegenerative diseases such as Alzheimer's disease (AD), and other dementias, Brain Cancer, Encephalitis, Epilepsy, Genetic Brain Disorders, Head and Brain Malformations, Hydrocephalus, Stroke, Parkinson's Disease, Multiple Sclerosis, Amyotrophic Lateral Sclerosis (ALS or Lou Gehrig's Disease), Huntington's Disease, Prion Diseases, and others. Inflammatory cytokines have been implicated in neuroinflammatory disorders such as Anxiety and Depression, and even childhood disorders such as ASD.

The term "nitrosative stress" is used to indicate the cellular damage elicited by reactive nitrogen species (RNS), including nitric oxide (NO) and its congeners peroxynitrite (OONO-). Here we are referring to iNOS as it relates to its intracellular up-regulation as is common in chronic infection. Free radicals are generated in the brain during normal intake of oxygen and to a greater degree, during infection. Oxidative damage is a likely outcome in chronic, low-grade infection in the brain because it is exposed to high oxygen concentrations—utilizing about one-fifth of the oxygen consumed by the body; contains relatively poor concentrations of antioxidants; is enriched in iron, which is a potent catalyst for oxidative species formation; and is rich in polyunsaturated fatty acids, which are themselves prone to oxidation.

It is widely accepted that Oxidative Stress (OS) increases as we age, and it can be considered an important age-dependent factor making the brain more susceptible to several neurodegenerative diseases such as Alzheimer's disease (AD), Parkinson's disease (PD), amyotrophic lateral sclerosis (ALS), and chronic infection. Several studies show markers of oxidative damage and neuroinflammation—such as glial activation, up-regulation of cytokines, lipid peroxidation, and protein and DNA oxidation—in the affected brain regions. Cytokine-stimulated microglia generate significant amounts of reactive oxygen and nitrogen species (RNS) leading to neurotoxicity. An age-dependent increase in reactive oxygen species (ROS) may be directly responsible for amyloid precursor protein (APP) cleavage to Aβ production resulting in sporadic AD.

Multiple sclerosis (MS) is an inflammatory, demyelinating disease that has both autoimmune and OS ties. Reactive oxygen species (ROS), leading to OS, generated in excess primarily by macrophages, have been implicated as mediators of demyelination and axonal damage in MS. ROS cause damage to cellular components such as lipids, proteins, and nucleic acids, thereby resulting in early cell death and subsequent immune responses against self-antigens as dead and dying cells become a major source of the self-antigens. This is true not just in MS but may be the etiology of Lupus, ALS, Chronic Lyme disease (CLD) and other neurological disorders with autoimmune components.

Let me summarize the pathogenesis due to toxic exposure this way:

1. Environmental factors such as toxins enter the CNS through damages in the BBB.
2. Toxins produce an oxidative stress (OS) by inducing early cell death, ROS, and subsequent self-tissue breakdown from dying and dead cells that builds up faster than can be carried away
3. The self-tissue build-up of apoptotic debris is recognized by microglial cells as antigens, which leads to up-regulation of pro-inflammatory cytokines in the CNS and creation of an autoimmune response.
4. A cycle of destruction ensues further as B-cells produce antibodies and T-cells destroy self-tissue

Similar pathology regarding the presence of infection may be explained:
1. Chronic, subclinical (often gram-negative) bacteria cross the BBB
2. Lipopolysaccharides (LPSs) from the bacteria attract a Th1 response from microglial cells.
3. As bacteria are destroyed, they release debris in the form of endotoxins that illicit further inflammatory responses from CNS microglial cells and the cytokines not only produce ROS and RNS but also further iNOS production continues neuronal destruction as bacteria pursue intracellular pathways of protection against immune responses.
4. Neuronal destruction takes place via two pathways: direct destruction as described above with autoimmune responses to the tissue itself and indirect destruction with oxidative stress.

Another factor propagating an autoimmune disorder in either of the above two scenarios is the roll of a faltered apoptotic response in the immune system itself. Normal programmed apoptosis in the immune system is *critical* for maintaining self-tolerance and preventing autoimmunity. Oxidative stress and/or chronic infection, coupled with an inhibited apoptotic process in lymphocytes or dendritic cells spells disaster!

When I write about apoptotic malfunctions, I'm usually using cancer in the same paragraph yet here, with defective dendritic cell apoptosis, we see resulting accumulation of and, chronic lymphocyte activation and systemic autoimmune manifestations with all sorts of different names. Fas (also known as Apo-1 and CD95) receptors have been suggested to control T cell expansion by triggering T cell-apoptosis. Other receptors are also being identified and though it is unclear why down-regulation of these receptors takes place, as in cancer, many possible mechanisms exist for their malfunction including the very toxin or infection in question.

Note: This same model can be interpolated with traumatic brain injury (TBI) patients as the inflammatory response in trauma mimics that of infection, especially in repetitive traumas.

Let's understand the infectious process better. In the case of gram-negative bacteria, which we're proposing to be the primary culprit in many cases, infiltration into the CNS requires damage to the BBB. This can be a closed system as the bacteria itself is perfectly capable of damaging endothelial lining and breaking the astrocyte border. Gram-negative bacteria have a peculiar cell membrane consisting of a polysaccharide chain and a lipid portion known as lipid A, collectively, we call this a lipopolysaccharide (LPS). Lipid A is hydrophobic in nature and is toxic in itself, however, the importance to the human immune system is what we are interested in as LPSs stimulate a strong Th1, T-cell response. As immune cells breakdown gram-negative bacteria, LPS is released; this LPS is known as an endotoxin.

LPSs then possess a unique ability to cause disease. Inflammatory cytokines recognize these remnants of bacterial cell walls as enemies and the endotoxins become antigens in an endless cycle of bacterial proliferation, immune stimulation, bacterial breakdown releasing LPS, immune stimulation against LPS endotoxins, renewed bacterial proliferation, renewed immune stimulation, excessive release of LPSs, increase up-regulation of destructive cytokines, as so on, as so forth. The patient is left with a progressive tissue, autoimmune disorder wherever the primary infection began and is given diagnoses such as Endothelial dysfunction (if the primary destruction is giving the patient heart symptoms), MS, AD, etc. if the infection expresses in the CNS, or cancer.

You see, if you simply recognize an inflammatory process and attempt to quench the inflammation, you increase the chronicity of the disorder and do little to help the patient! Below are the gram-negative bacteria that are responsible parties in such infectious cycles:

- Acetobacter - Acetic acid from ethanol and pose no threat to humans
- Borrelia – Spirochete from ticks commonly causing Lyme Disease and are common culprits causing neurological syndromes
- Bordatella – causing Pertussis
- Burkholderia – causing B cepacia common in Cystic Fibrosis patients. Due to their antibiotic resistance and the high mortality rate from their associated

diseases B. mallei and B psuedomallei are considered to be potential biological warfare agents, targeting livestock and humans

- Campylobacter – causing GI infections as a common food-borne infectious disease
- Chlamydia - Intercellular Parasite group causing STDs and "walking pneumonia". Is a common cause of endothelial disease
- Enterobacter – causing many UTI (urinary tract infections) and GI infections. There are some studies that reveal a sharp increase in Enterobacter species and subsequent endotoxin inflammation in the GI tracts of obese patients.
- Escherichia – (E. coli) found in normal GI tract flora yet imbalance causes many issues in certain species.
- Fusobacterium – contribute to a variety of disease including Gingivitis, Periodontal disease, Cancers of the GI tract, Ulcerative Colitis, and Endothelial disease (therefore BBB disruption)
- Helicobacter – possible the most prevalent of all gram-negative bacteria in humans, Helicobacter contributes to too many disease to list including Peptic Ulcer, Endothelial Disease, any Cancer, skin lesions, neurodegenerative disorders such as MS, AD, and ALS, and many autoimmune disorders.
- Haemophilus – causing H influenza, URI (upper respiratory infections), Epiglottitis, Meningitis, Otitis, etc.
- Klebsiella – causing Hemorrhagic pneumonia, UTI, skin infections, and soft tissue infections
- Legionella – causing the pneumonia of the Legionnaire's disease
- Leptospira – Spirochete causing leptospirosis, can cause a wide range of symptoms, some of which may be mistaken for other diseases. Some infected persons, however, may have no symptoms at all. Without treatment, Leptospirosis can lead to kidney damage, meningitis (inflammation of the membrane around the brain and spinal cord), liver failure, respiratory distress, and even death
- Neisseria – causing N gonorrhea, N meningitides
- Nitrobacter - Nitrogen fixing bacteria
- Proteus - causing Opportunistic UTI. About 10-15% of kidney stones are caused by alkalization of the urine by the action of the urease enzyme from Proteus
- Pseudomonas - causing Nosocomial infections (acquired at a hospital), common in burn patients, and Cystic Fibrosis patients
- Rickettsia - causing Rocky Mountain spotted fever
- Salmonella – causing typhus, Food poisoning
- Serratia - causing Opportunistic UTIs, Respiratory Infections
- Shigella - causing Dysentery
- Thiobacter - Sulfur reducing
- Treponema – Spirochete, T pallidum - causing Syphilis
- Vibrio – causing Cholera, GI disease usually associated with eating undercooked seafood.
- Yersinia – plague causing bacteria that, like Shigella, hides within host macrophages

Dr. Kevin Conners, Dr. Kelly Halderman

Treatment MUST be centered on correcting the cause. Infectious organisms MUST be dealt with or you (the practitioner) risk increasing the tissue destruction and actually worsening the patient's condition.

The difficulty in killing these diseases is threefold:

1) The problem with using direct-contact agents such as antibiotics is that the bacteria, in a micro-evolutionary attempt at survival, will morph its frequency to stay alive. This is why Legionella, for example, was the mystery of a 1976 American Legion convention killing 34 people and sickening 221 others. Was it a 'new' disease? Why are antibiotic-resistant bacteria the fear of hospital workers? It's not the fault of the antibiotics or even over-prescription; it is the resilience of the Bacteria, regardless of the circumstances, to morph its biological frequency to 're-create itself' one could say.

2) Using herbal stimulants, commonly prescribed by natural doctors and used by millions may do more harm than good. If the disorder has progressed to a Th1, pro-inflammatory process as described above, stimulation to the immune response will bring greater destruction of self-tissue! This is NOT a good idea!

3) Lab identification is extremely difficult as the chance that organism will show up in a blood test is highly unlikely. Gram-negative bacteria are insidious as many have the ability to hide intracellularly, entering the cell cytoplasm similar to strategies of certain virus – through cell membrane receptors. Here they evade immune destruction and are able to reproduce and create an ongoing cycle. The bacteria that remain extracellular remain in tissue where their death releases LPS endotoxin debris that creates the autoimmune process. Attempting solely to kill the bacteria with chemical agents (either antibiotics or herbal immune stimulators) will prove futile should the process have had any considerable amount of time to take hold.

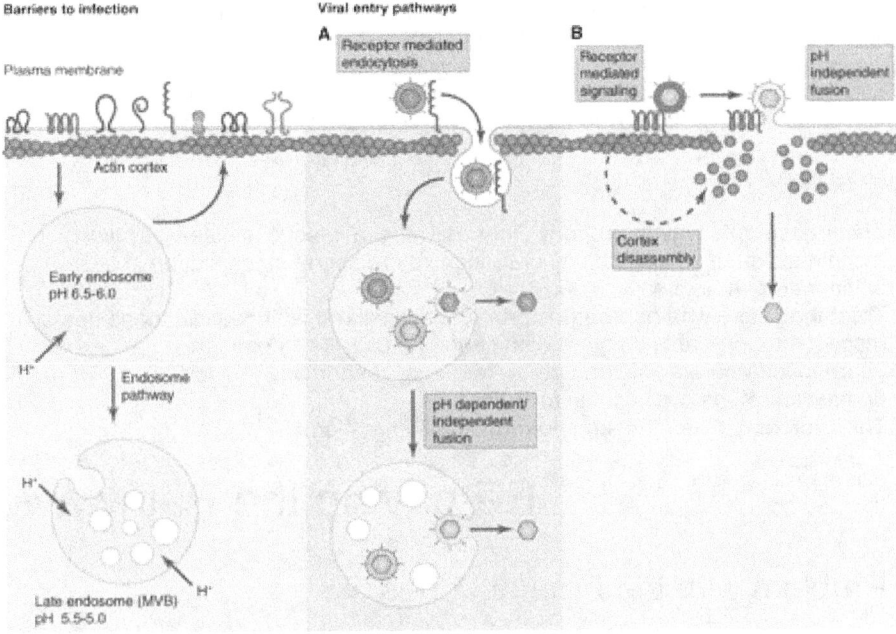

It is our recommendation that one must utilize frequency medicine in eradicating such intruders. This is the only way one can adequately account for both survival mechanisms employed by the bacteria – its constant micro evolutional form-change and its stealth-like ability to hide within the host's cells.

Chronic Lyme disease is the easiest example as the Borrelia bacteria can only be killed by antibiotics within a specific window of time prior to their invasion of cellular cytoplasm and forever hiding away from mainstream medical approaches. Another, Shigella flexneri, a bacterium that infects people through feces-contaminated food and causes severe diarrhea and vomiting, first attaches to and then penetrates *macrophages*—the very immune cells that are supposed to devour invading pathogens—as they patrol the intestines. Shigella multiplies inside the macrophage cells, where it is unchallenged by the immune system attempting to kill it like a bank robber escaping in the police car that is searching for him. Eventually, the infected macrophage dies and releases new bacteria that spread to and infect nearby epithelial cells and cause destruction of the intestinal tissue.

Another type of bacterium, Mycoplasma, composes a ubiquitous group of minute microorganisms that lack a cell wall. Of the seven species, which have been isolated from man, only Mycoplasma pneumonia (commonly known as walking pneumonia) has clearly established pathogenicity. Research continues to seek other possible disease relationships, since there are various animal diseases caused by mycoplasmas, which have counterparts among human illnesses of unknown cause. Cancer research has concentrated on mycoplasmas since many cancers have shown to possess a higher concentration of mycoplasma infection than normal tissue. M. Pneumonia can be associated with a wide spectrum of respiratory tract disease, including bullous myringitis, pharyngitis, tracheobronchitis, pneumonia, and other subclinical infections that can lead to autoimmune responses. Like their gram-negative counterparts, mycoplasmas are rarely diagnosed as the disease-causers that they are.

Bottom-line 'take home':

1. Either develop a way to properly diagnose stealth infectious diseases with techniques such as kinesiology or recognize the secret signs hidden in the inflammatory markers.
2. Treat the cause with appropriate pharmaceutical and Nutriceutical measures respecting a probable immune dominance (usually Th1 dominant).
3. Learn to incorporate Rife and other frequency technology to assist the destruction of the organism in question.
4. Then you may take measures to reduce inflammation.

Re-paving the Pathways

The Problem with the Frontal Lobes

As stated, Anxiety, Depression, OCD and the rest of the ASD's are primarily frontal lobe disorders. Imbalance between the two hemispheres, a failure of reciprocal communication, and typically a decrease frequency of firing of the right as compared to left may be the cause of the collective symptoms. Though there may be many reasons why this is occurring, from the emotional environment already discussed to the genetic predisposition to auto-immune responses to metabolic stimuli, correction of the imbalance must accompany the metabolic correction.

Elkhonin Goldberg, in his classis book "The Executive Brain" reverberates, "Frontal lobes are critical for every successful learning process, for motivation and attention. Today we are increasingly aware of subtle disorders afflicting both children and adults – attention deficit disorders (ADD) and attention deficit hyperactivity disorder (ADHD)…how they are caused by subtle dysfunction of the frontal lobes and the pathways connecting them to other parts of the brain."

Dr. Kevin Conners, Dr. Kelly Halderman

Frontal Lobe

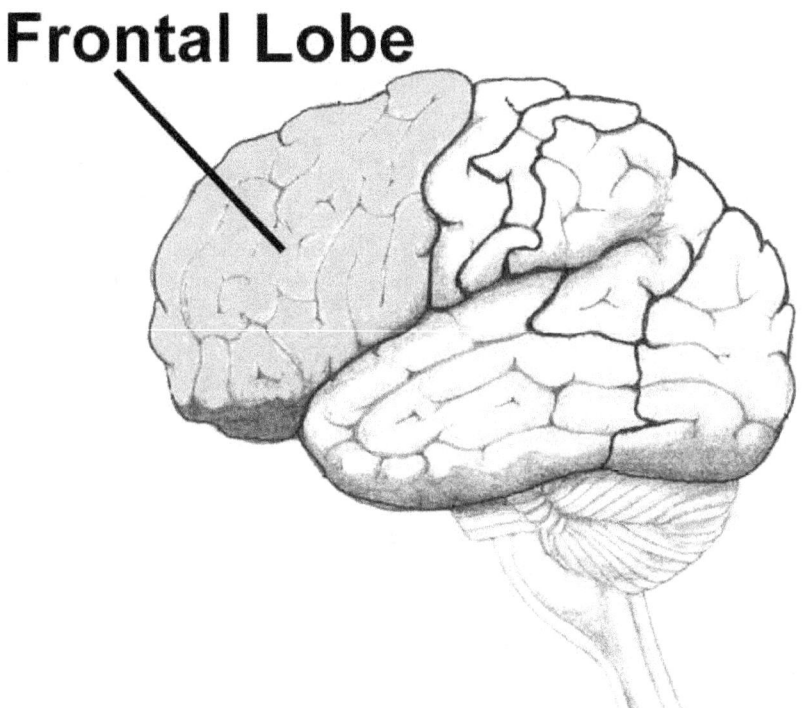

The frontal lobes are the executive of the brain, the CEO of all human function. They are concerned with all sophisticated operations of information processing, language processing, abstract thought and general reasoning. They are truly what make you human. Your dog does have frontal lobes but they are relatively small by comparison. Dogs receive less neuronal firing of the frontal cortex back onto the midbrain (the part of the brain responsible for instinctual function) and therefore are more governed by instinctual function. As much as I try to teach my German Sheppard NOT to bark at passersby or the squirrel at the feeder, she has a difficult time suppressing the instinctual protective features bred into her.

A properly functioning frontal cortex is what makes us human. It regulates movement, sorts all cognitive input, balances emotion responses, and decides on appropriate behavior. The most anterior portion (most frontal), is called the pre-frontal cortex. It is the conductor of the brain and is separated into three distinct gyri: the Dorso-Lateral gyrus, the Frontal-Orbital gyrus, and the Medial Anterior Cingulate.

Pre-Frontal Lobe Syndromes

Dr. Kevin Conners, Dr. Kelly Halderman
"The Musicians follow the Conductor"

Dorsi-Lateral (DL) Gyrus-
- Helps decide what is relevant
- Helps perspective, Helps sequence
- Helps attenuate, Helps categorize
- Helps sort, organize thoughts and future plans
- Gives emotional affect

Dysfunction or hypofunction:

Left DL Gyrus:
- Wrong data
- Learning issues
- Difficulty sorting info
- Planning difficulty
- Difficulty attenuating importance of data
- Difficulty sorting the outcomes of different data
- Mixing up data
- Inability to initiate and then to terminate an activity
- Difficult planning and changing a plan

Early Alzheimer's & Dementia are Frontal Lobe dysfunctions. The FL is the parent, or conductor that neuronally fires back on deeper brain centers, keeping them alive. The DL gyrus is essential in life drive – Subtle decrease in drive, initiative, and interest in the world around is a common early sign of Dementias.

Tests:
-Wisconsin Card Sorting Test
-Stroop test

Right DL Gyrus:
Similar/same as left plus an emotional charge to it or worse with data that has emotional impact/characterization

More severe → the more indifferent patient will be to the problem!

note: = OCD (commonly from a lack of inhibition to the DL Gyrus from the Basal Ganglion – a deep central portion of the midbrain), Mental Rigidity (they 'need' to fire the frontal lobe with OCD behaviors)
= Perseveration on things, actions, Field-Dependant behavior
= 'can't let things go', these OCD traits all stem from DL Gyrus problems

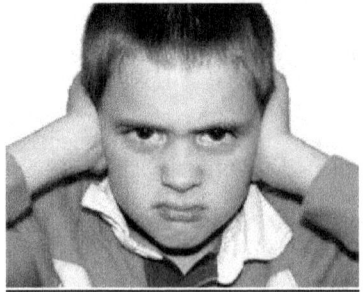

Frontal-Orbital Gyrus-
- Helps determine consequences of possible behavior

- Helps base decisions against outcomes = the voice of reason

Dysfuntion/hypofunction:
- Increased risk taker;
- impairment of insight,
- Lack of impulse control & foresight
- Increased asocial behavior
- Loss of inhibition of behavior (Tourette's spectrum – they 'need' to fire the FL with tics, verbal expression)
- Moral Agnosia, ability to KNOW right from wrong but inability to use this knowledge to regulate behavior

note: There can be an increased weight of consequences = Anxiety, lack of action, Panic Attacks

> Wizelsucht Syndrome – Drunken adolescent attitude – immature, self-absorbed personality. What was known as a 'pseudo-sociopath'.
> **Frontal-Orbital Gyrus = social maturity**
> = Inappropriately jocular, emotionally volatile, irritable, fractious, & impulsive.
> =ADD, ADHD, Asbergers, Autism-spectrum
> =Addictions, phobias, impulsive habits

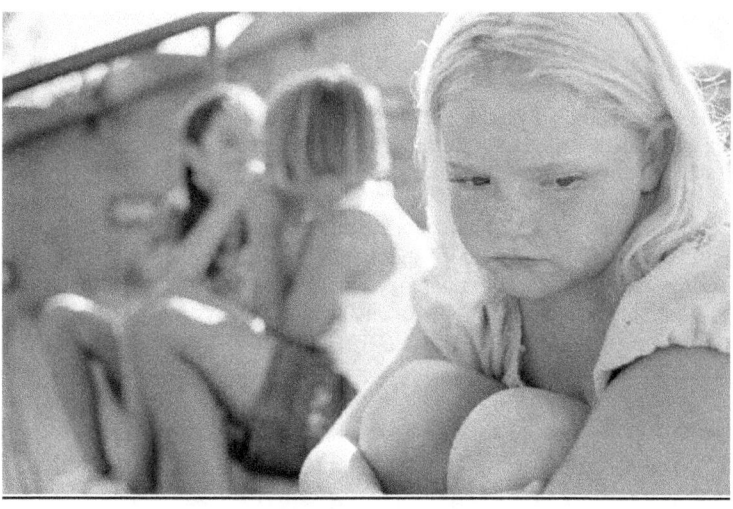

Medial Anterior Cingulate (MAC)
Helps base possible behaviors weighed against rewards

Dysfunction/hypofunction:
- No longer driven by the potential emotional rewards
- Akinetic, lack of 'tone' in personality, lack of emotion
- Lose perspective of emotional consequences

- Lose perspective of moral/ethical consequences
    - -lose compassion
    - -lose empathy
    - -pain of others doesn't bother them

Dysfunction/hyperfunction:
- Increase risk taker,
- Dangerous behavior,
- 'Forbidden' behavior
- Gravitate towards self-destructive behavior, sports, games
- Micturation (urination centers) area is next to MAP, therefore pt may have incontinence, bedwetting issues

The Pre-Frontal Cortex is the CEO of the Brain; it is the Conductor of the Orchestra. It is what makes us human, what separates us from the beasts. It is the stimulator of all that is good in the Brain and the inhibitor of all less desirable. The Pre-Frontal Cortex is what makes you, you!

Important Note:
Hypo/Hyper-firing of the brain is a **relative state** between Left & Right sides or different brain centers that a person experiences in Brain-Based Conditions. Most people with brain-based issues tend to fluctuate between states.

EG: OCD and Tourette's have their classical symptoms expressed as a 'hyper' state in the
There almost never exists a singular lesion manifesting in only one of the Pre-frontal Gyri. It is more complex, more subtle changes, commonly ignored or missed by the individual and their family. But, if caught early, serious, permanent changes may be averted!

Anxiety, Depression & Postpartum Depression Neurology

Postpartum depression (PPD) is a potentially debilitating disorder that develops in a significant and ever increasing percentage of women during the first year after giving birth. Women afflicted with PPD can even experience long-term consequences, including sadness, guilt, and despair and their offspring may be affected as well. Two biological systems that may play a significant role during the postpartum period are the immune system and the hypothalamic-pituitary-adrenal (HPA) axis. Dysregulation in either system individually or in their bidirectional interaction is associated with the development of PPD.

One particular observation has focused on studies revealing PPD women's regulation of the HPA axis components, adrenocorticotropic hormone (ACTH) and subsequent release of cortisol by the adrenals. While PPD women seem to have a normal spike of ACTH (the pituitary hormone that stimulates the release of cortisol) under stress conditions, there is a definite suppression in the adrenal response.

The action of CRH (CRH is secreted by the paraventricular nucleus (PVN) of the hypothalamus in response to stress) on ACTH (in pituitary) release is strongly potentiated by vasopressin that is also produced in increasing amounts when the hypothalamic paraventricular neurons are chronically activated. The end action of CRH is immunosuppression, suppression of detox pathways, and increase in release of glucose stores via the action of cortisol, CRH itself can heighten inflammation, particularly locally in the CNS, increasing the risk of neurogenic disorders.

Vasopressin stimulates ACTH release in humans and hence cortisol; its antagonist, oxytocin inhibits it. There is interesting research on oxytocin, thought of as the 'bonding' hormone because of its release in intimate moments that bring about the feeling of love, nurture, and connection; some believe that stimulating its production either through neuronal pathways, metabolic precursors, or direct supplementation of the hormone may help depressed and anxious patients. This also makes sense in PPD patients. If they have ramped-up ACTH pathways, suppression of the antagonistic oxytocin pathways will lead to the 'failure to bond' patterns common in PPD women.

Side note – common with many other frontal lobe disorder patients, including depression, anxiety, ADD/ADHD, can be increased ACTH pathways and subsequently suppressed oxytocin secretion. This can explain many of the symptoms found in these disorders including lack of bonding, difficulty in social situations, and general lack of empathy for others, etc.

ACTH release results in the release of corticosteroids from the adrenal that, subsequently, through mineralocorticoid and glucocorticoid receptors, exert negative feedback on direct brain pathways in the hippocampus, the pituitary and the hypothalamus. In Alzheimer's disease (AD) and major depression the HPA-axis is hyperactive. Increased production of vasopressin in depression may lead to increased plasma levels of vasopressin that have been related to an enhanced suicide risk. The increased firing activity of oxytocin neurons (possibly in an attempt to keep them alive) in the paraventricular nucleus (PVN) may be related to the eating disorders in depression and similar brain disorders.

You gain strength, courage, and confidence by every experience in which you really stop to look fear in the face. You are able to say to yourself, 'I lived through this horror. I can take the next thing that comes along.'
Eleanor Roosevelt

In depressed women, plasma levels of estrogen are usually lower and plasma levels of androgens are increased, while testosterone levels are decreased in depressed men. This is explained by the fact that both in depressed males and females the HPA-axis is increased in activity, parallel to a diminished HPG-axis (gonadal), while the major source of androgens in women is the adrenal, whereas in men it is the testes. Therefore it seems important to not only balance brain output to these structures but to look at metabolic disturbances as well.

Environmental toxic exposures include pesticides, most notably glyphosate (Roundup); industrial chemicals such as polybrominated diphenyl ether (PDBE) flame retardants (in all children's clothing), pthalates, bisphenol A (BPA – found in most plastics); neurotoxic metals such as mercury and aluminum (tooth fillings, vaccinations, many other things); and carcinogens such as dioxins. With 80,000 registered agents in the Toxic Substances Inventory, only 200 have been studied for human safety parameters. An important case series supported by the Environmental Working Group and the Red Cross examined umbilical cords, identifying 287 toxic chemicals, 217 of which are known neurotoxins! PDBE and BPA have been associated with adverse cognitive, endocrine and motor outcomes in children, and while ubiquitous, may represent a modifiable exposure in our immediate environment. We need to make better choices in purchases – you can find organic children's clothing. Even though these may be more expensive, demand will drive the prices downward.

A relatively recent discovery is the psycho-neuro-immunologic bridge—the kynurenine pathway (a tryptophan metabolite). The kynurenine: tryptophan ratio has been used as a marker of inflammation correlated with postpartum depressive behaviors and states. Inflammatory messengers, cytokines IL6 and TNF-alpha, have been demonstrated to be elevated in the cerebrospinal fluid of women at the time of their childbirth, who then presented with depression six weeks postpartum. Similarly, elevated levels of IL-1B predicted postpartum depressive symptoms. In the non-pregnant population, inflammatory underpinnings of depressive illness (cytokines, chemokines, reactive proteins, adhesion molecules) have been well-established, and anti-inflammatory interventions should be explored as these inflammatory agents result in a net decrease of serotonin, the neurotransmitter associated with a happier you.

Possible markers to check:

- Homocysteine

- CRP

- Fasting insulin/glucose

- HgA1C

- Vitamin D 25 OH and 1,25

- Methylmalonic acid

- TSH, free T3, free T4 and thyroid antibodies

- Celiac panel

- Methylenetetrahydrofolate reductase (MTHFR) genetic profile.

Dr. Kevin Conners, Dr. Kelly Halderman

Dementias

Dementia is not a specific disease but a term that describes a wide range of symptoms associated with a decline in memory or other cognitive skills severe enough to reduce a person's ability to perform everyday activities. Alzheimer's disease is the most common dementia and what is important to note is *any* dementia is NOT normal. It is important to note that early signs of cognitive decline spell one thing – brain inflammation. This is why we have questions on our New Patient intake forms like: Do you have brain fog, memory loss, forgetfulness, etc.?

Don't ignore the early onset signs of dementia as it is usually very gradual, and it is often impossible to identify the exact time it began. During the early phase of dementia, the person may:

- Appear more apathetic, with less sparkle; slight personality changes.
- Lose interest in hobbies or activities; appear more tired.
- Be unwilling to try new things; this is a big sign!
- Be unable to adapt to change.
- Show poor judgment and making poorer decisions than expected.
- Be slower to grasp complex ideas and take longer with routine jobs.
- Blame others for 'stealing' lost items.

> *Inaction breeds doubt and fear. Action breeds confidence and courage. If you want to conquer fear, do not sit home and think about it. Go out and get busy.*
> Dale Carnegie

- Become more self-centered and less concerned with others and their feelings.
- Become more forgetful of details of recent events.
- Be more likely to repeat themselves or lose the thread of their conversation.
- Be more irritable or upset if they fail at something.
- Have difficulty handling money and the decisions with it.

Imaging has a well-established place in the diagnostic work-up of a patient with possible Alzheimer's disease (AD) but remains a late-sign in diagnostic tools. Historically the role of imaging in a patient with cognitive impairment was limited to one of exclusion: namely to rule out a neoplasm, hematoma, hydrocephalus or other potentially surgically treatable causes and then just blame dementia. Although important, these conditions account for a tiny fraction of subjects with cognitive complaints. Unfortunately, a differential diagnosis in the dementias offers little hope anyways as treatment through traditional medicine seems dismal.

Diagnostically a large number of studies have shown that particular patterns of cerebral atrophy on structural imaging (MRI or CT) and hypo-metabolism on functional imaging (PET/SPECT) are associated with early Alzheimer's disease. Other functional tests may include standard neurological examination that reveals frontal lobe dysfunction;

Dr. Kevin Conners, Dr. Kelly Halderman
however, this is far from telltale for AD.

Functionally, AD is our most common dementing illness, characterized by premature synaptic and neuronal loss along with amyloid β (Aβ) plaques and tau tangles in the areas of the brain that are involved in memory consolidation, especially the limbic cortex including the hippocampus. This is why some have referred to AD as Diabetes Type 3. In a speech by Dr. Zetterberg, MD, PhD, from the Sahlgrenska Academy at the University of Gothenburg entitled, "Biomarkers for Alzheimer's Disease: Where are We," Dr. Zetterberg states, "Several novel therapeutics are being tested in clinical trials, but AD poses a number of challenges to the research community and pharmaceutical industry. How can we be sure that the memory-impaired individuals we are studying really have AD and how large is the influence on the symptoms of other disorders, such as cerebrovascular disease? How can we be certain that healthy controls do not have preclinical AD?"

Maybe the problem is that while medicine seeks ways to label a set of symptoms as early as possible, we are missing the point. Why are we not putting our effort into correcting early signs? I'll tell you why – traditional medicine doesn't know how! Millions of dollars pour in to organizations to 'find a cure' and yet the incidence of cancer and Alzheimer's disease continue to escalate. This debilitating neurodegenerative disorder, estimated to affect 5 million people in the USA alone, with incidence expected to increase fourfold over the next decade should be treated at early stages!

Here's a handy list from the Alzheimer's Association: Have you noticed any of these warning signs? Please list any concerns you have and take this sheet with you to the doctor.

1. Memory loss that disrupts daily life. One of the most common signs of Alzheimer's, especially in the early stages, is forgetting recently learned information. Others include forgetting important dates or events; asking for the same information over and over; relying on memory aides (e.g., reminder notes or electronic devices) or family members for things they used to handle on their own. What's typical? Sometimes forgetting names or appointments, but remembering them later.

2. Challenges in planning or solving problems. Some people may experience changes in their ability to develop and follow a plan or work with numbers. They may have trouble following a familiar recipe or keeping track of monthly bills. They may have difficulty concentrating and take much longer to do things than they did before. What's typical? Making occasional errors when balancing a checkbook.

3. Difficulty completing familiar tasks at home, at work or at leisure. People with Alzheimer's often find it hard to complete daily tasks. Sometimes, people may have trouble driving to a familiar location, managing a budget at work or remembering the rules of a favorite game. What's typical? Occasionally needing help to use the settings on a microwave or to record a television show.

4. Confusion with time or place. People with Alzheimer's can lose track of dates, seasons and the passage of time. They may have trouble understanding something if it is not happening immediately. Sometimes they may forget where they are or how they got there. What's typical? Getting confused about the day of the week but figuring it out later.

5. Trouble understanding visual images and spatial relationships. For some people, having vision problems is a sign of Alzheimer's. They may have difficulty reading, judging distance and determining color or contrast. In terms of perception, they may pass a mirror and think someone else is in the room. They may not recognize their own reflection. What's typical? Vision changes related to cataracts.

6. New problems with words in speaking or writing. People with Alzheimer's may have trouble following or joining a conversation. They may stop in the middle of a conversation and have no idea how to continue or they may repeat themselves. They may struggle with vocabulary, have problems finding the right word or call things by the wrong name (e.g., calling a watch a "hand clock"). What's typical? Sometimes having trouble finding the right word.

7. Misplacing things and losing the ability to retrace steps. A person with Alzheimer's disease may put things in unusual places. They may lose things and be unable to go back over their steps to find them again. Sometimes, they may accuse others of stealing. This may occur more frequently over time. What's typical? Misplacing things from time to time, such as a pair of glasses or the remote control.

8. Decreased or poor judgment. People with Alzheimer's may experience changes in judgment or decision-making. For example, they may use poor judgment when dealing with money, giving large amounts to telemarketers. They may pay less attention to grooming or keeping themselves clean. What's typical? Making a bad decision once in a while.

9. Withdrawal from work or social activities. A person with Alzheimer's may start to remove themselves from hobbies, social activities, work projects or sports. They may have trouble keeping up with a favorite sports team or remembering how to complete a favorite hobby. They may also avoid being social because of the changes they have experienced. What's typical? Sometimes feeling weary of work, family and social obligations.

10. Changes in mood and personality. The mood and personalities of people with Alzheimer's can change. They can become confused, suspicious, depressed, fearful or anxious. They may be easily upset at home, at work, with friends or in places where they are out of their comfort zone. What's typical? Developing very specific ways of doing things and becoming irritable when a routine is disrupted.

Rapidly Progressing Dementia

Though most dementias develop slowly, allowing an unhurried evaluation, Rapidly Progressing Dementia (RPD) is different. A careful history alone will usually detect dementia secondary to medication use or chronic neural degeneration and routine laboratory assessments help to eliminate metabolic conditions that can cause dementia including anemia, electrolyte imbalance, liver or kidney failure, thyroid disease, toxicity, and vitamin B12 deficiency. The majority of slowly progressive dementias are secondary to Alzheimer's disease (AD), although there is an increasing recognition of non-AD dementias, including frontotemporal dementia (FTD), subcortical ischemia vascular disease (SIVD), Lewy body dementia (DLB), and other parkinsonian dementias such as cortical basal degeneration (CBD).

Prion diseases, such as Creutzfeldt-Jakob disease (CJD), occur when prion protein, which is found throughout the body but whose normal function isn't yet known, begins folding into an abnormal three-dimensional shape. This shape change gradually triggers prion protein in the brain to fold into the same abnormal shape causing a rapid decline in brain function. The most notable prion dementia is Infectious CJD, or what is known as mad-cow disease.

RPDs develop subacutely over weeks to months. As most dementing conditions take years to progress to death, RPD can be quickly fatal. A helpful differential diagnostic approach to dementia, highlighting neurodegenerative, toxic/metabolic, infectious, autoimmune, neoplastic, and other conditions to consider is listed below. As many types of conditions can cause all dementias as well as RPD can progress quickly, it is helpful to have a systematic approach to diagnosis.

I learned that courage was not the absence of fear, but the triumph over it. The brave man is not he who does not feel afraid, but he who conquers that fear.
Nelson Mandela

The Addicted Brain

I personally know physicians who, despite all their knowledge of destruction of neural tissue with alcohol consumption, continue to consume mass quantities on a more than regular basis. We've all seen pictures of individuals continue to smoke through a tracheotomy tube after a laryngectomy for cancer; and, despite loss of employment, health, family and life-threatening complications of disease, many people continue to drink alcohol or take drugs even when doing so yields depression and misery rather than pleasure.

These examples highlight the central question of any addiction: Why do we continue destructive behavior even when we know it is highly destructive and what happens in the brain to cause an addicted person to seemingly lose control of their will? Neuroscientists have identified specific pathways that fire with use of every known drug of abuse, and they have specified common neural areas that are affected by almost all such drugs. Researchers have also identified the major receptors for virtually every chemical addition, as well as the natural ligands (that which are supposed to connect to) for most of those receptors. In addition, they have explained many of the biochemical cascades within the cell that follow receptor activation by drugs.

Research has also begun to reveal major differences between the brains of addicted and non-addicted, regardless of the substance. Virtually all drugs of abuse have common effects, either directly or indirectly, on a single pathway deep within the brain. This pathway, the mesolimbic reward system, extends from the ventral tegmentum to the nucleus accumbens, with projections to areas such as the limbic system and the orbitofrontal cortex. Stimulation of this system appears to be a common element in what keeps drug users taking drugs – what is called the addictive cycle. This activity is not unique to any one drug; all addictive substances affect this circuit in some way or another.

There is much evidence that the dopaminergic system is the major substrate of reward and reinforcement for both natural rewards and addictive behavior. This is known as the mesolimbic pathway; they are dopamine driven pathways that begin in the ventral tegmental area, an area in the mesencephalon of the midbrain important in cognition, motivation, orgasm, drug addiction, intense emotions relating to love, any behavioral addiction and several psychiatric disorders. This mesencephalic area connects to the limbic system via the nucleus accumbens (NAc), the amygdala, and the hippocampus as well as to the medial prefrontal cortex.

The NAc is involved in responding to the motivational significance of stimuli, and the dorsal striatum (major input station of the basal ganglia system) is involved in the learning and execution of behavioral sequences that permit an effective response to those cues. Addictive drugs as well as reinforced addictions increase the levels of synaptic dopamine in the NAc;

Opiates represent a partial exception to the central role of dopamine. Although opiates can produce reinforcement by dopamine release, they can also interact directly with opioid receptors on NAc neurons. Under normal circumstances, this dopaminergic circuit is a crucial substrate for the rewarding and reinforcing effects of positive natural stimuli associated with survival, such as food and reproductive opportunities.
I find it fascinating that these striatal connections are best known for planning and action of movement pathways (to the motor cortex) but also involved in a variety of other cognitive processes involving executive function (from the pre-frontal cortex), such as working memory. In humans, the striatum is activated by stimuli associated with reward, but also by aversive, novel, unexpected, or intense stimuli (typically from the RIGHT prefrontal cortex). Think about this; addictions may be linked as a survival mechanism in an individual's attempt to keep the prefrontal cortex alive!

Whether related to addiction or survival, actions that increase synaptic dopamine in this brain 'reward' circuitry tend to be repeated. Understanding that addiction is, at its core, a brain pathway disorder, changing the function of said pathways means that a major goal of treatment must be either to "un-pave" the hyper-stimulated pathways and "re-pave" the inhibitory tracts. The powerful control over behavior exerted by addictions results from the brain's inability to distinguish between the activation of the reward loop by naturally rewarding activities, such as healthy eating habits, healthy sex lives, healthy levels of alcohol consumption, and by the overconsumption, over-use, and over-indulgence as seen in addictive behavior. This inability to 'put on the brakes' is a lesion in the above described pathway from and to the prefrontal cortex. Remember, the prefrontal cortical firings onto midbrain centers are inhibitory; absence of said connections equals the absence of inhibition of behavior.

Therapy for Addictions

Whenever we pursue attractive goals, the neurochemical dopamine is released. Dopamine is absorbed by brain structures responsible for narrowed attention, effortful action, and above all, desire—the visceral thrust that motivates goal seeking. When addiction sets in—whether to drugs, booze, cigarettes, sex, gambling, food, or something else, what starts out as an episode of pleasure (or relief) begins to control the dopamine pump. Soon, dopamine release is determined by the anticipation of getting more, and the overlapping neural networks of desire and intentional action are increasingly tuned to that singular goal – the thrill of the hunt. The problem with addictions is that those specific networks also become less and less sensitive to other goals. This is why therapy designed at firing prefrontal cortical pathways is best for unwinding the addictive personality.

Again, as addictive behavior is reinforced (repeated), areas of the cortex that represent what's important and valuable (the addiction) become four-lane freeways. More and more synapses are devoted to the addictive behavior: thinking, reminiscing, planning, imagining—constructing intricate strategies for getting, all pave the path, not just the behavior itself. That is, thinking about drinking alcohol fires the same pathway as the act itself! At the same time, cortical regions responsible for cognitive control and self-monitoring become less effective; it's as if they become dirt pathways until they are eventually overgrown and turn back into forest.

So, treatment must begin with removing any obstacles to the pathway and then firing those neurons as if you are reconstructing lost trails into interstate systems. This is the beauty of Neurofeedback and daily brain-based therapies. Also consider neurotransmitter support with nutritional precursors and homeopaths. Most importantly, find a competent functional neurologist who will assess you as described in this book.

You want Biomarkers?

Diseases of the central nervous system are found in patients with severe hyperhomocysteinemia (HHcy). Levels greater than 8.0 may indicate early inflammation and shouldn't be ignored. Epidemiological studies show a positive, dose-dependent relationship between mild-to-moderate increases in plasma total homocysteine concentrations (Hcy) and the risk of neurodegenerative diseases, such as Alzheimer's disease, vascular dementia, cognitive impairment or stroke. HHcy is a surrogate marker for B vitamin deficiency (folate, B12, B6) and a neurotoxic agent and should be checked and treated by every primary physician.

Other lab tests should include those spelled out under our section on vascular/BBB disruption, liver pathway evaluation (such as an organic acid profile), hormone testing in the form of a 24-hour cortisol test, extended female hormone panel and male hormone panel, heavy metal and toxicity testing, and intestinal dysbiosis testing. There are many

An excuse for lack of early treatment in neurodegenerative diseases such as Alzheimer's, Parkinson's and Huntington's is that by the time symptoms appear, significant brain damage has already occurred-and currently there are no treatments that can reverse it. This is absolutely false! In most cases, the first symptoms are excused as patients justify the lesion and doctors, with no known cure, wait until symptoms escalate to the point of granting a diagnosis. A team of SRI International researchers has demonstrated that measurements of electrical activity in the brains of mouse models of Huntington's disease could indicate the presence of disease before the onset of major symptoms. The findings published as, "Longitudinal Analysis of the Electroencephalogram and Sleep Phenotype in the R6/2 Mouse Model of Huntington's Disease," in the July 2013 issue of the neurology journal *Brain*, published by Oxford University Press.

SRI researchers led by Stephen Morairty, Ph.D., a director in the Center for Neuroscience in SRI Biosciences, and Simon Fisher, Ph.D., a postdoctoral fellow at SRI, used electroencephalography (EEG), a noninvasive method commonly used in humans, (see chapter on Neurofeedback) to measure changes in neuronal electrical activity in a mouse model of Huntington's disease. Identification of significant changes in the EEG prior to the onset of symptoms would add to evidence that the EEG can be used to identify biomarkers to screen for the presence of a neurodegenerative disease. Further research on such potential biomarkers might one day enable the tracking of disease progression in clinical trials and could facilitate drug development.

"EEG signals are composed of different frequency bands such as delta, theta and gamma, much as light is composed of different frequencies that result in the colors we call red, green and blue," explained Thomas Kilduff, Ph.D., senior director, Center for Neuroscience, SRI Biosciences. "Our research identified abnormalities in all three of these bands in Huntington's disease mice. Importantly, the activity in the theta and gamma bands slowed as the disease progressed, indicating that we may be tracking the underlying disease process."

There is much research justifying the use of EEG screening for early brain changes. Until now, most investigations of EEG in patients with neurodegenerative diseases and in animal models of neurodegenerative diseases have shown significant changes in EEG patterns only after disease symptoms occurred. Its evidence in other neural dysfunctions is clearly demonstrated as well.

Since the landmark UCLA study (published in the American Journal of Drug and Alcohol Abuse in 2005), other reputable institutions have replicated their outcomes using the same protocols. Substance abusers have been shown to have similar dopamine receptor abnormalities. EEG testing reveals that the outcomes are always consistent if not better than the original UCLA results: 77 percent of participants who receive neurofeedback in conjunction with a 12-Step program remain abstinent at 12 months, compared to 44 percent of those who didn't receive neurofeedback, but who stayed in treatment longer.

Dr. Kevin Conners, Dr. Kelly Halderman

Neurofeedback testing, called a Brain Map, can be an early biomarker for neurodegenerative diseases as well as all neuroinflammatory disorders. Though we would always suggest a complete neurological and metabolic workup, such an easy scan as a Brian Map could be a lifesaver if abnormalities are found and subsequently corrected.

Typically, following the completion of EEG evaluation, a protocol is generated determining what sort of treatment will be most helpful for the patient. In general, Beta is provided for clients who have either under arousal of the left or right hemispheres, disrupting one's ability to focus and concentrate. EEG training of the beta wave at a different frequency supports calming, relaxation and objectivity. A combination of neurofeedback and metabolic treatments creates overall stability of brainwave activity and is particularly helpful for individuals with long-term mental health issues, chronic substance use disorders, early degenerative disease, ADD/ADHD, Anxiety, Depression, head injuries and a history of mental illness in their family origin.

"The literature, which lacks any negative study of substance, suggests that EEG biofeedback therapy should play a major therapeutic role in many difficult areas. In my opinion, if any medication had demonstrated such a wide spectrum of efficacy, it would be universally accepted and widely used. "
- Frank Duffy, MD, Neurologist, Head of the Neuroimaging Department and of Neuroimaging Research at Boston Children's Hospital, and Harvard Medical School Professor

There is really no excuse for not detecting brain disorders long before justifying a named disease; most doctors just don't know what to look for. Believe me, when I graduated, I learned every neurological test and every pathology but I had no idea what each test told me from a functional perspective. This is the beauty of functional neurology and functional medicine. The negative is that it takes years and tens of thousands of extra dollars beyond medical school loans to master this and few doctors are willing to 'go back to school' after decades of school.

Diagnosing Brain Conditions

The mnemonic VITAMINS is often useful for summarizing some of the major categories of etiologies of ALL brain symptom patients not just dementia. Doctors may find this helpful in assessing their patients and patients may help their doctors dig deeper by following this plan:

V = Vascular

As previously discussed in the section on blood-brain barrier disruption, the vascular system is the first thing a doctor should consider in all brain-symptom patients. A breakdown of the vascular endothelial barrier is the first consideration in all chronic disorders and he we shall refer to chronic as any patient with symptoms of 2-3 months progression.

Dr. Kevin Conners, Dr. Kelly Halderman

Depending on the location, strokes can present as rapidly progressive dementia and rapid onset symptomology. Large vessel occlusions can cause microangiopathic thromboses producing global cerebral ischemia, resulting in an encephalopathy. Autoimmune conditions in the CNS can and most likely will cause vasculitis and can mimic stroke/TIA acute symptoms. A vasculitis may be limited to the central nervous system without any systemic or peripheral nervous system signs or may initially present as a systemic disorder with accompanying fever, weight loss, rash, neuropathy, and other organ involvement. Urinalysis may contain red cells as a sign of renal involvement. Oxidative stress on vascular tissue may cause both chronic and acute infiltration of inflammatory chemicals that can lead to symptoms.

There may be signs of a hemolytic anemia in a rapidly failing patient. A basic blood screen may include, ESR, CRP, ANA, RF, with other possible functional testing but primary CNS vasculitis patients typically have normal non-specific tests, such as ESR, ANA and CRP. Chronic CNS symptoms involving vascular systems primarily involve intimal lining infiltration. As in cardiac patients, cerebral patients can exhibit arterioles that have luminal occlusions due to inflammation blistering under the intimal cell layer that bulge into the blood flow. For the sake of our analysis, let's concentrate on that which will most commonly be seen.

1. Assess stroke symptomology – we will not enter in to this discussion in this book but it suffices to say that in any acute case, this is the first assessment to be made.
2. Every patient with chronic brain issues as discussed in this book, with the possible exception of traumatic brain injuries (TBI), can assume they have a cerebral vascular breakdown. I believe that is a fair assumption given an understanding of both endothelial and astrocyte barriers. Every clinician should progress with treatment of the patient under that assumption and will have a much happier patient if causes are corrected, barriers are rebuilt and pathways are reconnected. See the section on BBB and possible supplementation for healing.
3. Vasculitis, the inflammation of tiny vessels in the brain has long been discussed as possible etiologies in migraines. Commonly associates with some connective tissue diseases such as systemic lupus erythematosus (SLE) rheumatoid arthritis, use of drugs such as amphetamine, cocaine and heroin, and certain forms of cancer (particularly lymphomas, leukemia and lung cancer). More commonly, patients are told their condition is idiopathic (which is Latin for "I have no idea"). There is always a reason why.

Doctor, we must think of acute vascular inflammatory episodes in light of understanding vascular cellular dynamics. In order for contraction and dilation to take place (and this is what we are talking about), the intimal cells open their doors (receptors) to chemicals that allow smooth muscle contraction. The tiny smooth muscle layer under the intimal lining is under direct control and direction of the intimal lining, and, more specific, the receptors.

The AT2 (angiotensin 2) receptor allows smooth muscle contraction, and the nitric oxide (NO) receptors aide in relaxation. From a neurological perspective, think of AT2 as under the control of the Sympathetic nervous system as it is responsible for increasing blood pressure and flow, and the NO system as part of the Parasympathetic nervous system tied to dilation, decreased blood flow and pressure. Neither one is "good" or "bad" so let's understand that first; it is all about balance!

The question we must ask is: What causes imbalance? There are only three possible physiological causes of imbalance within this cellular system – acute inflammation, oxidative stress, and autoimmune response. The causes of these are literally infinite and discussed ad nauseam in this book but include toxicity, vaccinations, heavy metals, excitotoxins, foods, etc.

I = Infectious

For most of the major neurological diseases including Alzheimer's, Parkinson's, multiple sclerosis, narcolepsy, schizophrenia, the cause, as far as traditional medicine is concerned, is elusive. We may know the neurons involved, for instance that Parkinson's is caused by a loss of substantia nigra dopamine neurons, and narcolepsy is caused by loss of hypothalamic hypocretin neurons, but why these cells are lost remains a mystery to most. Biotoxins must be considered! A growing understanding of the biology of the hundred or so viruses and other biotoxins that are known to infect the brain is finally raising the interest of researchers to the possibility of causation of a number of more subtle neurological conditions.

Infections of the brain are less common than that of other organs because biotoxins should not be able to penetrate the blood brain barrier. Therefore, most systemic infections do not enter the brain. See my reasoning of step one – fix the barriers! Biotoxins that do cross damaged barriers can cause neurological problems due to a number of mechanisms including lytic effects on brain cells (cytomegalovirus, h. pylori, lyme), induced apoptosis (vesicular stomatitis virus, VSV), or secondary damage due to release of glutamate (an excitatory neurotransmitter), release or even destruction of other neurotransmitters, destructive attacks on neural cell bodies, DNA, and other inducers of further brain damage.

The region in the brain that is infected plays a key role in the type of resulting dysfunction as many biotoxin infiltrations will remain local to an area. Limbic infections will manifest a completely different syndrome than infections of motor or sensory systems however; there is commonly an expression of global dysfunction possibly due to resultant inflammation and/or cytokine release by microglial cells. Infections such as cytomegalovirus, rubella, and lymphocytic choriomeningitis virus cause serious abnormalities if the developing brain is infected, and depending on the site and age of fetal infection, can generate distinct symptoms such as deafness, blindness, epilepsy, hydrocephalus, and/or reduced IQ in a manner directly related to what part of the brain was infected. The age of the infected individual also plays a large role in some infections; different biotoxins such as h. pylori, which is usually chronic, subacute (and usually un-diagnosed) can cause neurologic dysfunction at every stage of life. West Nile Virus and Chronic Lyme (CLD), are more likely to cause neurological problems in the

Dr. Kevin Conners, Dr. Kelly Halderman

that can be progressive and destructive. MS is due to an autoimmune attack on oligodendrocytes, but what is the antigen that sparks the attack? it might be initiated by a transient viral infection of those cells. While no single biotoxin has consistently been associated with MS, viruses such as measles and/or other biotoxin that sometimes infect oligodendrocytes have been associated with the disease.

Viral infections can also generate neurological problems years or decades after the initial infection, even after the infection is long dead. Chicken pox, a herpes virus, can remain latent in neurons for decades, to return years later as shingles when the live virus is regenerated from its latent genome – crazy stuff! The frequency of the organism is imprinted on the patient's DNA. The herpes simplex genome can also remain latent in peripheral neurons (particularly in the ganglions) for long periods before the active, replication-competent virus is regenerated, and travels down the axon to once again infect the periphery (example – cold sores). Some viruses leave a latent imprint on the brain that causes neurological dysfunction decades after the virus has been eliminated from the brain by the immune system. Postpolio syndrome is one example. Humans that have had symptoms of poliomyelitis and recovered can again show symptoms, such as weakness of affected limbs, 30–40 years later.

It gets worse: these same biotoxins and substances of vaccinations that were exposed to the patient years or decades ago, not only can resurface causing neurological symptoms with microglial immune responses but can cause cellular disruptions in apoptotic and replication cycles which we call cancer!

Bottom line – ignore these at your own risk!

How does one assess for these?

1. CSF (cerebral spinal fluid) testing would be typically recommended by traditional medicine but would routinely reveal false negative for obvious reasons: there is no infectious organism in the CSF. CSF inspection solely checks CSF.
2. MRI/CT evaluations will reveal late-stage infectious outcomes such as cyst or abscess formation common to trichinosis, as well as acute infectious processes exhibiting inflammation such as encephalitis.
3. Blood testing can show abnormalities in white counts but this is not indicative of cerebral infections. Blood testing for antibodies to brain tissue may be affective, as in testing for cerebellar antibodies but again, it will reveal an autoimmune disorder but not the antigen in question, which may be a number of different things other that an infectious organism.
4. Kinesiology testing, though controversial and demands a practitioner with years of experience is still the most accurate at detecting specific infectious causes particularly the chronic, subclinical causes of insidious inflammation. Finding a practitioner is the greatest challenge. We have had numerous seminars training doctors from around the world and hold clinical rounds for practitioners wanting to learn more. If you are a licensed practitioner, contact our office or visit our website and register for an upcoming seminar or our practitioner pages giving more information on functional diagnoses.

Doctors, cognitive dysfunction is a common neurological syndrome of infectious causation although usually a late complication. Syphilis, for example, can present with rapid progression, particularly in immune-compromised patients. Lyme disease is a systemic infection with the spirochette, Borrelia burgdorferi and numerous co-infections, which is usually transmitted to people from a tick bite. Neurological manifestations are common in Lyme disease, including cranial nerve palsy, meningitis, polyradiculopathy, depression, psychosis, and dementia. It is important to differentiate acute versus chronic Lyme as acute should immediately be treated with an antibiotic, typically doxycycline. Although rapidly progressive dementia caused by Lyme disease has been reported, it is chronic Lyme (CLD) that usually causes slow yet progressive neurological symptoms. CLD no longer responds to antibiotic therapy as it literaly morphs its frequency (not unlike antibiotic resistant bacteria) into a viral-like pathogen that can hide intracellularly in both the CNS and systemic cells.

Subacute sclerosing panencephalitis (SSPE) is a chronic CNS infection from the virus that causes measles and is still occurs in individuals from countries where measles infections are common. It typically occurs in children, but can occur in adults. Worse, people having been vaccinated for measles (MMR) may carry the DNA encode and exhibit CNS symptoms accordingly. Patients can develop the same progressive dementia, seizures (focal and/or generalized), myoclonus, ataxia, rigidity, and visual disturbances. All these symptoms can vary in degree and pattern to confuse both patient and doctor as to etiology leaving most patients misdiagnosed and mistreated!

Finally, infectious organisms are common antigens in autoimmune (AI) reactions everywhere in the body, including the CNS. If the Ai disorder leaves one in a Th1 dominant state (see my book on AI disease, "Help, My Body is Killing Me..."), it makes it extremely challenging to treat as most recommended pathogen 'killers' are Th1 stimulators. There is much to learn, I know, but a greater understanding yields a better success rate with the most challenging cases, and these are the ones I love!

T = Toxic-metabolic conditions

Metabolic causes of brain pathway disruption include everything from vitamin deficiencies, endocrinologic disturbances (which we'll discuss separately) and everything that we've discussed earlier in this book. Vitamin deficiencies (usually from taking synthetic compounds) can result in significant neurologic deficits, including cognitive impairment.

Pellagra ("rough skin") is due to niacin deficiency and is classically described as "the three Ds" - dermatitis, diarrhea and dementia. Niacinamide, or nicotinamide, is what we find in food and commonly call niacin. Niacin can have side effects, but these are minimal when coming from plant food sources. Synthetic Vitamin B3 – Nicotinic acid is created using coal tar, ammonia, acids, 3-cyanopyridine, and formaldehyde. It is less absorbable and has risks of side effects, which ironically include niacin deficiency syndromes. Niacin deficient causes abnormalities of the skin and gastrointestinal tract, as well as peripheral neuropathy, myelopathy and cognitive dysfunction. With a careful history, the dementia of pellagra is typically found to be insidious, not rapid. Niacin deficiency should be considered in patients with nutritional deficiency, such as alcoholics and patients with anorexia nervosa, as well as in those taking isoniazid (used to treat tuberculosis). Finding nicotinic acid metabolites in the urine make the diagnosis easy but, this is just another reason to use a whole-food B-complex on every most patient.

Deficiency of thiamine (Vitamin B1), a necessary cofactor in oxidative metabolism, can cause Wernicke's Encephalopathy, which classically presents as a triad of ophthalmoparesis (with vertical and/or horizontal nystagmus), ataxia and memory loss. The thalamic involvement on MRI can appear similar to that seen in CJD and cause the patient similar symptoms, which are quite severe. Thiamin is a water soluble vitamin created by plants and bound to phosphate. Digestion releases the thiamin using specialized enzymes. Synthetic Vitamin B1, Thiamine mononitrate, or thiamine hydrochloride, is again made from coal tar, ammonia, acetone, and hydrochloric acid. It is crystalline in structure (like many synthetic vitamins), unlike plant-based vitamins. Crystals in our blood stream cause damage and mineral accumulation where it isn't needed, like joints. All patients with brain symptoms should be screened for Vitamin B12 deficiency.

Numerous toxins can cause brain issues. Exposure to heavy metals, such as arsenic, mercury, aluminum, lithium, and lead can lead to cognitive decline, particularly following acute exposure. Even minerals, again usually consumed in wrong forms through supplements can cause toxicity. Iodine and iron would be prime example of this. I've had too many patients to count that have presented taking large doses of elemental iron (usually ferrous sulfate) and iodine, thinking they are helping their anemia or thyroid respectively. Even calcium, commonly seen in supplements as calcium carbonate are incorrect forms of nutrients. It is literally like eating dirt! Remember, plants take nutrients in dirt and convert them to the appropriate form for us. We then eat the plant, not the soil!

Manganese toxicity, found usually in miners, can present with significant Parkinsonism. Bismuth is a metal used to treat gastrointestinal disorders (Pepto Bismol), principally peptic ulcer disease and diarrhea. Bismuth intoxication, typically caused by overdosing (and usually prolonged exposure –meaning frequent use) on bismuth containing products can cause a disorder mimicking CJD (mad-cow disease). Patients initially manifest with apathy, mild ataxia, headaches, which progresses to myoclonus, dysarthria, severe confusion, hallucinations (auditory and visual), seizures, and, in severe cases, even death.

We've already discussed excitotoxins, possibly the most common brain toxin as they readily cross even healthy blood-brain barriers. Pesticides, herbicides, and household cleaners, even chemical in shampoo and soap can all lead to toxic encephalopathy. The wide variety of slow-onset symptoms, which can include memory loss, personality changes/increased irritability, insidious onset of concentration difficulties, involuntary movements, fatigue, seizures, arm strength problems, and depression, usually lead people to never suspect a toxic source. Neurobehavioral effects of occupational exposure to organic solvents among those working with chemicals are common. The condition may also be referred to as substance-induced persistent dementia due to the cognitive decline commonly seen. Acute intoxication symptoms include lightheadedness, dizziness, headache and nausea, and regular cumulative exposure to these toxic solvents over a number of years puts the individual at high risk for developing brain disorders that usually receive a different named diagnosis.

Common toxins, used daily, can cause cancer. A recent study of pediatric brain tumors in Los Angeles County, California involving mothers of 224 cases, investigated the risk of household pesticide use from pregnancy to diagnosis. Risk was "significantly elevated" for prenatal exposure to flea/tick pesticide "particularly among subjects less than 5 years old at diagnosis" suggesting exposure to chemicals at younger ages cause greater harm. Frontline, and other similar brands of flea/tick applications boast season-long prevention to your dog or cat with a simple liquid applied to their back. Just think of the toxic exposure not just to your pet that will die in several years given a shorter life expectancy and the cause of death will probably be blamed on old age and not cancer, but the exposure to everyone in contact with your pet. The damage to the brain of your pet, your children and yourself from these poisons is simply unnecessary. Most people could deal with their dog being a little loopy but we just cannot ignore the dangers to humans.

It doesn't take a rocket scientist to figure out that there'll be a difference in toxic load of 10-pound child compared to a 200-pound man when it comes to household chemical exposures. Vaccinations are another concern with toxins especially if the child has damaged/lagging liver detoxification pathways and a compromised blood-brain barrier. But still we think injecting egg or chicken protein, viruses, Neomycin, Polymyxin, Gentamycin antibiotics, Thimerosal, Betapropiolactone, Nonoxynol, Octoxinol, Formaldehyde, Polysorbate 80, and Triton X-100 is GOOD for a 6-pound infant?

Research points to the toxic effects of not only active but also *inactive* ingredients found in everyone's cupboard – hazards that can affect the central nervous system, reproductive systems and other vital bodily systems. Consumers often don't have the time or know where to go to find important information about the products they use, but they must become educated. To make matters worse, the information is often presented in highly scientific language that may be difficult to interpret or hidden (legally I might add) behind inclusive phrases like "other natural and artificial flavorings". But there are a growing number of consumer-friendly resources that can help us sort through all of this information and understand what we need to know to make the best possible choices for our families with regard to household cleaners, disinfectants and polishes.

For starters, the three essential categories into which most of the hazardous ingredients in household cleaning products fall are:

1.   **Carcinogens**– Carcinogens cause cancer and/or promote cancer's growth.
2.   **Endocrine disruptors** – Endocrine disruptors mimic human hormones, confusing the body with false signals. Exposure to endocrine disruptors can lead to numerous health concerns including reproductive, developmental, growth and behavior problems. Endocrine disruptors have been linked to reduced fertility, premature puberty, miscarriage, menstrual problems, challenged immune systems, abnormal prostate size, ADHD, non-Hodgkin's lymphoma and certain cancers.

3. **Neurotoxins** – Neurotoxins alter neurons, affecting brain activity, causing a range of problems from headaches to loss of intellect. Excitotoxins fit into this category.

Reading labels

People may find it time-consuming to research all of the ingredients in the cleaning products under the kitchen sink and foods that they buy. In general however, product warning labels can be a useful first line of defense. Cleaning products are required by law to include label warnings if harmful ingredients are included. From safest to most dangerous, the warning signals are:

Signal Word	Toxicity if swallowed, inhaled or absorbed through the skin*
Caution	One ounce to a pint may be harmful or fatal
Warning	One teaspoon to one ounce may be harmful or fatal
Danger	One taste to one teaspoon is fatal

*For a 180-pound male

Even products with a cautionary label, it should be pointed out, may present health risks if used improperly or with repeated exposures over time. Good ventilation and skin barriers are very important when using any over-the-counter cleaning product.

We are exposed to countless chemical ingredients in daily life that may be harmful to our health – too numerous to outline here and beyond the scope of this article. Consumers should know of some general categories of chemicals that should be avoided, however. The following list is not all-inclusive.

Pesticides. One of the most counter-intuitive health threats is that of products that disinfect. Common sense tells us that killing household germs protects our health. However disinfectants are pesticides, and the ingredients in pesticides often include carcinogens and endocrine disruptors. Pesticides are fat-soluble, making them difficult to eliminate from the body once ingested. Pesticides, including disinfectants, may also include alkylphenol ethoxylates (APEs).

APEs. APEs act as surfactants, meaning they lower the surface tension of liquids and help cleaning solutions spread more easily over the surface to be cleaned and penetrate solids. APEs are found in detergents, disinfectants, all-purpose cleaners and laundry cleansers. They are also found in many self-care items including spermicides, sanitary towels and disposable diapers. APEs are endocrine disruptors.

Formaldehyde. Formaldehyde is commonly known as a preservative. Many people do not know that it is also a germicide, bactericide and fungicide, among other functions. Formaldehyde is found in household cleaners and disinfectants. It is also present in nail polish and other personal care products. Formaldehyde is a carcinogen.

Organochlorines. Organochlorines result from the combination of hydrogen and carbon. Some types are highly deadly, such as DDT. OCs are bioaccumulative and also highly persistent in the environment. OCs are present in pesticides, detergents, degreasers and bleaches. OCs are also present in drycleaning fluids. OCs are carcinogens and endocrine disruptors.

Styrene. Styrene is a naturally occurring substance derived from the styrax tree. Styrene is most commonly used in the manufacture of numerous plastics including plastic food wrap, insulated cups, carpet backing and PVC piping. Styrene is also found in floor waxes and polishes and metal cleaners. Styrene is a known carcinogen as well as an endocrine disruptor. Exposure may affect the central nervous system, liver and reproductive system.

Phthalates. Phthalates are most commonly used in the manufacture of plastics. Phthalates are also used as carriers for perfumes and air fresheners and as skin penetration enhancers for products such as moisturizers. These chemicals are classified as inert and as such no product-labeling requirements exist for phthalates. They are endocrine disruptors and suspected carcinogens. Phthalates are known to cause hormonal abnormalities, thyroid disorders, birth defects and reproductive problems.

Volatile Organic Compounds (VOCs). VOCs are emitted as gases suspending themselves in the air. VOCs include an array of chemicals, some of which may have short- and long-term adverse health effects, and are present in perfumes, air fresheners, disinfectants and deodorizers. VOCs commonly include propane, butane, ethanol, phthalates and/or formaldehyde. These compounds pose a variety of human health hazards and collectively are thought to be reproductive toxins, neurotoxins, liver toxins and carcinogens.
Diagnosing toxic exposure is difficult without utilizing a technique such as Kinesiology. Blood testing can reveal acute exposure but once the toxin penetrates the blood-brain barrier, it typically is no longer circulating in the blood. Tissue samples will reveal toxicity but again, this isn't very practical and I have yet to find a volunteer to give me a brain sample.

Getting rid of toxic substances typically requires chelation therapy. A chelator is simply a known nutraceutical that binds to inorganic substances to carry them out of the body. EDTA is the most widely known chelator. EDTA was first synthesized in the late 1930s in Germany and its first documented clinical use in lead poisoning was first reported in 1952, when Michigan battery factory workers were discovered to be suffering from lead poisoning. They were treated with EDTA and coincidentally those patients who had coronary artery disease and angina had also a lessening of those symptoms following treatment. This prompted the first studies to discover other therapeutic effects of EDTA. The first study of EDTA in occlusive vascular disease (clogged arteries) was stopped due to lack of immediate results. However, it was resumed after patients reported subsequent improvements in symptoms. It was found that maximum benefits occurred approximately three months following a course of treatment. More than 500,000 people have been treated with chelation therapy in the United States alone, without a single reported incident of renal failure or death since 1960 and yet cardiovascular disease is still the most common cause of death in the US. So, why isn't it used more? Maybe it's because the pharmaceutical companies can't own the patent.

Here we are discussing chelation's approach to toxins. There are many substances that act as chelators of toxins in the body. Though I test patients for the specific product and dosage that is best for them, I'll list my favorites, in no particular order here:

1. Gama Detox - Premiere Research Labs
2. IP6 – I use Hope Science
3. DMSA – several sources
4. EDTA suppositories – several sources
5. Modified Citrus Pectin
6. Cilantro
7. Chlorella

Reputable labs produce most of the above products and have other beneficial components added to enhance detoxification. I highly suggest that you do NOT attempt chelation without professional help and NEVER do any detoxification without supporting liver detox pathways!

A = Assess Hormone Function

We cannot discuss the brain without addressing hormonal balance as hormones affect the balance of serotonin, dopamine, GABA, and norepinephrine, the brain neurotransmitters responsible for stabilizing our moods, and connecting nerve pathways. Estrogen fluctuations (in both sexes), can cause brain serotonin to drop to low levels, which severely impacts function. Without adequate levels of serotonin in your brain, you may experience agitation, irritability, anxiety, depression, and loss of inhibition of angry and impulse. It's a vicious cycle in women because low serotonin levels inhibit the ability of a woman's ovaries to produce adequate amounts of estrogen.

Traumatic brain injuries (TBIs) may cause damage to the hypothalamus and/or pituitary gland, which are the brain's generators responsible for regulating the body's hormones. The effects of pituitary and hypothalamus injury are many and varied because of the huge amount of hormones which can be affected as these are the master stimulators of all the glands. Some symptoms are similar to the more common effects of brain injury and that is another reason why the problem may be underdiagnosed.

Examples of overlapping symptoms are:

Depression
Sexual difficulties, such as impotence and altered sex drive
Mood swings
Fatigue
Headaches
Vision disturbance
Other symptoms include:

Muscle weakness
Reduced body hair
Irregular periods/loss of normal menstrual function

Dr. Kevin Conners, Dr. Kelly Halderman

Reduced fertility
Weight gain
Increased sensitivity to cold
Constipation
Dry skin
Pale appearance
Low blood pressure/dizziness
Diabetes insipidus

It is an error to think of hormone balance simply in terms of female cycles and menopause. Both sexes, at any age, experience ill effects of poor hormonal control. Located just behind and between the eyes, deep in the brain is the hypothalamus. It is bordered laterally by the optic tracts and temporal lobes and sits directly below the thalamus. It contains a series of differentiated nuclei that connect it with the rest of the brain and with the endocrine system.

The periventricular axon system in the hypothalamus contains axons that connect the hypothalamus with the brainstem and thalamus. Some periventricular axons communicate to the anterior pituitary and secrete releasing hormones where they control secretion of prolactin, thyrotropin, corticotropin, growth hormone, gonadotropic hormones, and prolactin. Other periventricular axons, from cells in the supraoptic and paraventricular nuclei that produce oxytocin or vasopressin, pass directly through the pituitary stalk to the posterior pituitary gland, where their terminals secrete these hormones into the general circulation.

The lateral hypothalamic axon system runs to the lateral hypothalamic area, serving to connect the more medial nuclei with the forebrain above, and with the brainstem below. The medial nuclei of the hypothalamus regulate fluid and electrolyte balance, body temperature, and sexual hormones. The brain's biological clock, the suprachiasmatic nucleus, is also at this level, sitting just above the optic chiasm, as do neurons that are critical for secreting melatonin and causing sleep. The middle third of the hypothalamus contains the nuclei that regulate feeding, hunger, energy metabolism, stress responses, and coordinate wake-sleep cycles.

Since the hypothalamus sits at a crossroads in the brain, receiving direct sensory inputs from the smell, taste, visual, and somatosensory systems, it may be considered the inter-communicator between the brain and the endocrine system. It also receives sensations for such things as blood temperature, blood sugar, mineral levels, and feedback loops for a variety of hormones. Thus the hypothalamus receives sensory inputs necessary to detect challenges in both the internal and external environments and enables one to adapt to life.

The hypothalamus receives inputs from frontal lobe areas, especially the hippocampus, amygdala, and cingulate cortex. Remember, these structures form the limbic lobe that drive a wide range of emotional responses associated with emotional expression (changes in heart rate, blushing/flushing, hair standing on end, etc.) are mediated by the hypothalamus.

Dr. Kevin Conners, Dr. Kelly Halderman

In summary, the importance of the hypothalamus is threefold. First, it regulates the internal milieu of electrolyte concentrations and osmolality, glucose and other fuels, and body temperature, maintaining homeostasis. Secondly, it helps the body deal with large and unpredictable alarms of outside dangers that require a change in behavior and physiology. The responses can include resetting various setpoints (e.g., increase in body temperature and blood pressure), as well as endocrine adjustments (such as cortisol and adrenaline release when under threat). Lastly, the hypothalamus helps anticipate daily events that are triggered by the external day-night cycle. We all have predictable times for feeding, drinking, sleeping, and sexual behavior. All of these are regulated by the circadian timing system in the brain that both the hypothalamus and hippocampus largely control.

From a neurological perspective, firing into the cerebellum will greatly affect the hypothalamus and hence, all hormone function. And remember, the cerebellum is the most vascular of brain structures and therefore, most susceptible to autoimmune and inflammation. Treatment hint: brain-based therapy aimed at cerebellum and frontal lobe function can go a long way in balancing hormones!

> *"Like sand on a beach, the brain bears the footprints of the decisions we have made, the skills we have learned, the actions we have taken."*
> -Sharon Begley, Train Your Mind, Change Your Brain

A holistic understanding of hormone balance cannot leave the gut out in the cold. Recent research has found, for example, that tweaking the balance between beneficial and disease-causing bacteria in our gut dramatically alters our brain chemistry. It goes both ways as the brain can also exert a powerful influence on gut bacteria; as many studies have shown, even mild stress can tip the microbial balance in the gut, making the host more vulnerable to infectious disease and triggering a cascade of molecular reactions that feed back to the central nervous system.

Symbiotic gut bacteria also produce hundreds of neurochemicals that the brain uses to regulate both basic physiological processes and mental processes such as learning, memory and mood. For example, gut bacteria manufacture about 90 percent of the body's supply of serotonin, which influences both mood and GI activity.

M = Malignancies
Several primary and secondary malignancies can cause an acute or subacute cognitive disorder. Three malignancies that often present as dementias, and present with varied abnormalities on MRI, are primary CNS lymphoma (PCNSL), intravascular lymphoma, and lymphomatoid granulomatosis. Any of the primary brain tumors can present with CNS symptoms with a sudden onset of headaches, dizziness, seizures, change in speech, vision or hearing, nausea or vomiting, sudden loss of memory, etc.

This book is not meant for an in-depth discussion on cancer, but functional medicine and functional neurology is fully capable to deal with the effects of space occupying lesions in the brain. A proper functional exam will reveal areas needing support and

Dr. Kevin Conners, Dr. Kelly Halderman

brain-based therapy as well as neurofeedback can greatly improve the patient's outcomes.

I = Injuries (TBI)

Traumatic Brain Injury (TBI) is classified below as to severity. Unlike more severe TBIs, the disturbance of brain function from mild TBI (MTBI) is related more to dysfunction of brain metabolism (what the trauma does to the brain chemistry) rather than to structural injury or damage. These are what will be seen by most physicians and should be understood by parents alike as these MTBIs are the repetitive microtraumas that bring symptoms of early cognitive decline years or decades later. The current understanding of the underlying pathology of MTBI involves a paradigm shift away from a focus on anatomic damage to an emphasis on neuronal dysfunction involving a complex cascade of ionic, metabolic and physiologic events. Clinical signs and symptoms of MTBI such as poor memory, speed of processing, fatigue, and dizziness result from this underlying neurometabolic cascade. (See CDC website)

Though there are several bedside tests that can be done at the scene of injury, at home after an event, or in a doctor's office, the Glasgow Coma Scale below is a simple way to classify an injury. It is based on a 15 point scale for estimating and categorizing the outcomes of brain injury on the basis of overall social capability or dependence on others. The test measures the motor response, verbal response and eye opening response with these values:

I. Motor Response
6 – Obeys commands fully
5 – Localizes to noxious stimuli
4 – Withdraws from noxious stimuli
3 – Abnormal flexion, i.e. decorticate posturing
2 – Extensor response, i.e. decerebrate posturing
1 – No response

II. Verbal Response
5 – Alert and Oriented
4 – Confused, yet coherent, speech
3 – Inappropriate words and jumbled phrases consisting of words
2 – Incomprehensible sounds
1 – No sounds

III. Eye Opening
4 – Spontaneous eye opening
3 – Eyes open to speech
2 – Eyes open to pain
1 – No eye opening
The final score is determined by adding the values of I+II+III.
This number helps medical practitioners categorize the four possible levels for survival, with a lower number indicating a more severe injury and a poorer prognosis:

Dr. Kevin Conners, Dr. Kelly Halderman

Mild (13-15):
A traumatic brain injury (TBI) can be classified as mild if loss of consciousness and/or confusion and disorientation is shorter than 30 minutes. While MRI and CAT scans are often normal, the individual has cognitive problems such as headache, difficulty thinking, memory problems, attention deficits, mood swings and frustration. These injuries are commonly overlooked. Even though this type of TBI is called "mild", the effect on the family and the injured person can be devastating.

Other Names For Mild TBI
- Concussion
- Minor head trauma
- Minor TBI
- Minor brain injury
- Minor head injury

Mild Traumatic Brain Injury is:
- Most prevalent TBI
- Often missed at time of initial injury
- 15% of people with mild TBI have symptoms that last one year or more.
- Defined as the result of the forceful motion of the head or impact causing a brief change in mental status (confusion, disorientation or loss of memory) or loss of consciousness for less than 30 minutes.
- Post injury symptoms are often referred to as post concussive syndrome.

Common Symptoms of Mild TBI
- Fatigue
- Headaches
- Visual disturbances
- Memory loss
- Poor attention/concentration
- Sleep disturbances
- Dizziness/loss of balance
- Irritability-emotional disturbances
- Feelings of depression
- Seizures

Other Symptoms Associated with Mild TBI
- Nausea
- Loss of smell
- Sensitivity to light and sounds
- Mood changes
- Getting lost or confused
- Slowness in thinking

These symptoms may not be present or noticed at the time of injury. They may be delayed days, weeks, months or even years before they appear. The symptoms are often subtle and are often missed by the injured person, family and doctors because they "look normal" and often have little dysfunction in spite of not feeling or thinking normal. This makes the diagnosis easy to miss. Family and friends often notice changes in behavior before the injured person realizes there is a problem. Often the frustration at work or when performing household tasks may bring the person to seek medical care.

Moderate Disability (9-12):
- Loss of consciousness greater than 30 minutes
- Physical or cognitive impairments which may or may resolve
- Benefit from Rehabilitation

Severe Disability (3-8):
- Coma: unconscious state. No meaningful response, no voluntary activities

Vegetative State (Less Than 3):
- Sleep wake cycles
- Aruosal, but no interaction with environment
- No localized response to pain

Persistent Vegetative State:
- Vegetative state lasting longer than one month

The Centers for Disease Control published a handy 'pocket card' for patients that have experienced TBIs:

What to Expect Once You're Home from the Hospital

Most people with a concussion recover quickly and fully. During recovery, you may have a range of symptoms that appear right away, while others may not be noticed for hours or even days after the injury. You may not realize you have problems until you try to do your usual activities again. Most symptoms go away over time without any treatment. Below is a list of some of the symptoms you may have:

- Thinking/Remembering
- Difficulty thinking clearly
- Feeling slowed down
- Trouble concentrating
- Difficulty remembering new information

Physical
- Headache
- Balance problems
- Blurred vision
- Dizziness
- Nausea or vomiting
- Lack of energy
- Sensitivity to noise or light

Emotional/Mood

- Irritability
- Nervousness
- Sadness
- More emotional

Sleep
- Sleeping more than usual
- Sleeping less than usual
- Trouble falling asleep

How to Feel Better
- Get plenty of rest and sleep.
- Avoid activities that are physically demanding or require a lot of thinking.
- Do not drink alcohol.
- Return slowly and gradually to your routine.
- Ask a doctor when it is safe to drive, ride a bike, or operate heavy equipment.

WHEN TO RETURN TO THE HOSPITAL
Sometimes serious problems develop after a head injury. Return to the emergency department right away if you have any of these symptoms:
- Repeated vomiting
- Worsening or severe headache
- Unable to stay awake during times you would normally be awake
- More confused and restless
- Seizures
- Difficulty walking or difficulty with balance
- Difficulty with your vision
- Any symptom that concerns you, your family members, or friends

N = Neurological – assessing the patient's pathways
Learning how to do a proper neurological examination is necessary for any physician. Learning how to interpret such an exam is for the 'big boys'. Sorry, I mean no offence to my colleagues that do not understand functional neurology but, no second thought, yes I do. Having taken hundreds of hours of Carrick seminars (www.carrickinstitute.com) and completed American Functional Neurology Institute with Dr. Andy Barlow, I highly recommend doctors study functional neurology prior to taking patients described in this book. It is like going back to medical school; unfortunately for patients, most doctors know nothing about that which we speak because of the former statement.

We have already covered enough neurology in this book to turn most non-doctors off so we'll go no deeper here except to state again that a medical neurologist will know nothing about functional neurology. Understanding HOW to do neurological tests and understanding what they MEAN is similar to the difference between being able to read Greek and being able to fully converse with an Athenian.

S = Systemic

Dr. Kevin Conners, Dr. Kelly Halderman

Inflammation elsewhere in the body sharply affects the blood-brain barrier. One study showed that injecting rats with inflammatory cytokines, interleukin-1 beta (IL-1 beta), interleukin-2 (IL-2), interleukin-6 (IL-6) and tumor necrosis factor-alpha (TNF-alpha) directly affected the permeability of the blood-brain barrier (BBB). The cerebral regional blood volumes appeared significantly lower in the rats injected with IL-6 (a Th2 cytokine) than in the control animals, but markedly increased following TNF-alpha (a Th1 cytokine) administration. This suggests that patients with systemic Th1 dominant autoimmune disorders may both damage the BBB and vasodilate cerebral microvessel endothelium and those with Th2 dominant disorders both damage BBB and vasoconstrict the cerebral microvessel endothelium.

Following episodes of immune, Th1 responses, proinflammatory cytokine levels in liver and serum typically return to basal levels within a day, whereas brain proinflammatory cytokines remain elevated for long periods. IL-10, an anti-inflammatory cytokine is reduced in brain by ethanol and LPS, while brain proinflammatory cytokines remain increased, whereas liver IL-10 is increased when proinflammatory cytokines have returned to control levels. Activation of brain microglia indicated by morphological changes, reduced neurogenesis and increased brain expression of COX-2 pathways. Alcohol consumption is a perfect example of an induced Th1 response inducer.

Peripheral cytokines both damage and penetrate the blood-brain barrier. There is abundant evidence that inflammatory mechanisms within the central nervous system contribute to cognitive impairment via cytokine-mediated interactions between neurons and glial cells. Peripheral immune cells also activate microglial immune responses. Cytokines mediate cellular mechanisms of cognition (e.g., cholinergic and dopaminergic pathways) and can modulate neuronal and glial cell function to facilitate neuronal regeneration or neurodegeneration.

A general dysregulation in immunological functioning is considered a hallmark of the aging process – though NOT normal. Increasing age has been associated with changes in serum balances of various cytokines. Apparently, IL-6 levels seem to increase with advancing age in various 'healthy populations'. Since IL-6 also causes osteoclastic activity, it is no wonder osteoporosis is common. Remember, what is 'common' should never be considered 'normal'. This is just another reason for the astute clinician to regulate their patient's immune system and why all osteoporotic patients should be evaluated for elevated IL-6 levels!

As such, it appears that increases in IL-6 represent a common outcome in aging in general and should be evaluated. The age-associated rise in IL-6 may also play a role in thymic atrophy and the suppression of thymopoiesis during aging. In addition, age-related increases in TNF-alpha and TNF receptors have been demonstrated in blood. The cause of this age-related cytokine dysregulation is unclear and could include normal homeostatic responses and other disease processes. My opinion is that many people have undiagnosed, subclinical Th2 dominant autoimmune disorders that lead to the high incidence of Th2 related diseases as we age; Cancer and Cardiovascular Disease are predominately Th2 dominant disorders!

One possible mechanism of this Th2 dominance in aging is suggested by findings that dehydroepiandrosterone (DHEA) inhibits IL-6 secretion. Thus, an age-related increase in IL-6 could also be due to a loss of tonic inhibition by DHEA as levels of this adrenal hormone decrease those of advancing age that exhibit adrenal fatigue, common in elderly.

We've discussed toxins at length but can't forget elevated glucose levels affecting brain and BB function as well. According to the Mayo Clinic, diabetes is considered a risk factor for vascular dementia as it can damage blood vessels in the brain. This form of dementia is often caused by reduced or blocked blood flow to the brain. But researchers from Germany now say that even those without diabetes who have high blood sugar levels may be at risk for impaired memory skills.

In the word recall test, the researchers found that remembering fewer words was linked to higher blood sugar levels. They break this down, stating that an increase of 7 mmol/mol of a glucose marker called HbA1c correlated with recalling two fewer words. Explaining their findings, Agnes Flöel, of the Charité University Medicine in Berlin and study author, told *Medical News Today*: "Clinically, even if your blood sugar levels are 'normal,' lower blood sugar levels are better for your brain in the long run with regard to memory functions as well as memory-relevant brain structures like the hippocampus. Scientifically, we were able to shed further light on the mechanisms mediating these effects. DTI-based (diffusion tensor imaging) measurements demonstrated that not only volume of the hippocampus, but also microstructural integrity is lower if blood sugar levels are higher."

Other Considerations

Functional and dissociative neurological symptoms have been given many different names over the years. Many people have been given labels have been considered 'psychiatric patients', which is based on the idea that the symptoms are 'all in the mind'. Psychological factors are often important to look at in relation to functional and dissociative neurological symptoms but the symptoms are not 'made up'. Most experts believe that these symptoms exist at the interface between the brain and mind, between neurology and psychiatry, which is why it is difficult when people ask "is it neurological or psychological?" In truth, it is always both, as there is no separation between hard pathways of function and emotional pathways of thoughts and feelings.

The follow list of labels does not make easy reading , but, upsetting as it may be to see some of these terms, it may help you to know about them.

Conversion Disorder - is a term made popular by Sigmund Freud and used in a standard US classification system of psychiatric disorders (DSM-IV). It refers to an idea that patients are 'converting' their mental distress in to physical symptoms. Conversion disorder refers to symptoms of weakness, movement disorder, sensory symptoms and non-epileptic attacks but has been expanded to mean any neurologic disorder that traditional medicine is unable to explain. The principle of "conversion" is something that may apply to a small minority of patients but there is little experimental evidence for the idea in the majority of patients.

Non-Organic - is a term doctors use for symptoms which are not due to identifiable disease or definable cause (at least to the extent of their knowledge). It implies the problem is purely psychological.

Psychogenic - is a term quite frequently used to describe these symptoms, especially dissociative seizures and movement disorders. Again it implies that the problem is purely psychological.

Psychosomatic - has come to mean the same as psychogenic although its original meaning was to describe the way in which the body affected the mind as well as psychological processes affecting the body

Somatization - suggests that the person has physical symptoms because of mental distress. The arguments here are the same as those for 'conversion disorder'. Somatization Disorder describes a situation where someone has a lifelong pattern of physical symptoms which are not due to disease.

> *"Half of what medical schools teach is wrong; the hard part is figuring out which half."*

While the emotional component to every illness must be investigated, we believe that, especially in long-standing conditions, several questions must be answered:

1. What will I have to 'give up' in order to get better? By this we must investigate things that we are currently holding (like addictions to substances and foods) as well as emotional ties that bind us (like freedom from responsibilities).
2. What areas in my life require change? I have encountered numerous patients that may even cry in my treatment room over the anguish of their current state yet they refuse to make lifestyle changes to save their life.
3. What responsibilities am I trying to avoid? In every case, even cancer cases, tough questions like this need to be addressed.
4. Are there any benefits to this disease? Are there any secondary 'gains' to continued sickness? Do I get the attention that I've longed for my entire life? Is this disease bringing me the pity, the devotion, the response from others that I missed from an absent parent?

Personal reflection is essential and honesty is crucial. No one should be ashamed if there are emotional components to their illness; it's normal. Facing these patterns head-on is the only way to overcome any disease and finding a safe place and friend to confide in is important.

Conclusion
This section was mainly for the clinician but can help direct the patient to proper care. The bottom line is that patients with brain-based problems should have a complete evaluation that aims at finding the cause. Arriving at a diagnosis is worthless. To give a collection of symptoms a Latin name does little to help the patient.

Dr. Kevin Conners, Dr. Kelly Halderman

Helpful Questionnaires

Grade each question on a scale of 1-5; (5 being the most troublesome, 1 being less of a problem)

Right Cortical Delay/Deficiency:

Clumsiness and an odd posture.	
Poor coordination	
Not athletically inclined and has no interest in popular childhood participation sports	
Low muscle tone – muscles seem kind of floppy	
Poor gross motor skills, such as difficulty learning to ride a bike, and/or runs and or/ walks oddly	
Repetitive/stereotyped motor mannerisms (spins in circles, flaps arms)	
Fidgets excessively	
Poor eye contact	
Walks or walked on toes when younger	
Poor spatial orientation – bumps into things often	
Sensitivity to sound	
Confusion when asked to point to different body parts	
Poor sense of balance	
High threshold of pain	
Likes to spin, go on rides, swing, motion	
Touches things compulsively	
A female interested in makeup and jewelry	
Does not like the feel of clothing on arms or legs	
Doesn't like being touched or to touch things	
Prefers bland food	
Does not notice strong smells such as burning wood, popcorn, cookies baking	
Avoids foods because of the way it looks	
Doesn't enjoy eating and not even interested in sweets	
Extremely picky eater	
Spontaneously cries and/or laughs and has sudden outbursts of anger or fear	
Worries a lot and has several phobias	
Holds on to past "hurts"	
Has sudden emotional outbursts that appear over reactive and inappropriate to the situation	
Experiences panic and/or anxiety attacks	
Sometimes displays dark or violent thoughts	
Face lacks expression; doesn't exhibit much body language	
Too uptight; cannot seem to loosen up	
Lacks empathy and feelings for others	
Lacks emotional reciprocity	
Often seems fearless and is a risk taker	
Logical thinker	
Often misses the gist of a story	
Always the last to get a joke	
Gets stuck in set behavior; can't let it go	
Lacks social tact and/or is antisocial and/or socially isolated	

Dr. Kevin Conners, Dr. Kelly Halderman

Poor time management is always late	
Disorganized	
Has a problem paying attention	
Is hyperactive and/or impulsive	
Has obsessive thoughts or behaviors	
Argues all the time and is generally uncooperative	
Exhibits signs of an eating disorder	
Failed to thrive as an infant	
Mimics sounds or words repeatedly without really understanding the meaning	
Appears bored, aloof, and abrupt Considered strange by other children	
Inability to form friendships	
Has difficulty sharing enjoyment, interests, or achievements with other people	
Inappropriately giddy or silly	
Acts inappropriately in social situations	
Talks incessantly and asks the same question repetitively	
Has no or little joint attention, such as the need to point to an object to get your attention	
Didn't look at self in mirror as a toddler	
Poor math reasoning (word problems, geometry, algebra)	
Poor reading comprehension and pragmatic skills	
Misses the big picture	
Very analytical	
Likes "slapstick" or obvious physical humor	
Is very good at finding mistakes (spelling)	
Takes everything literally	
Doesn't always reach a conclusion when speaking	
Started speaking early	
Has tested for a high IQ, but scores run the whole spectrum; or IQ is above normal in verbal ability and below average in performance abilities	
Was an early word reader	
Is interested in unusual topics	
Learns in a rote (memorizing) manner	
Learns extraordinary amounts of specific facts about a subject	
Is impatient	
Speaks in a monotone; has little voice inflection	
Is a poor nonverbal communicator	
Doesn't like loud noises (like fireworks)	
Speaks out loud regarding what he or she is thinking	
Talks "in your face" – is a space invader	
Good reader but does not enjoy reading	
Analytical; led by logic	
Follows rules without questioning them	
Good at keeping track of time	
Easily memorizes spelling and mathematical formulas	
Enjoys observing rather than participating	
Would rather read an instruction manual before trying something new	
Math was often the first academic subject that became a problem	
Has lots of allergies	

Rarely gets colds and infections	
Has had or has eczema or asthma	
Skin has little white bumps, especially on the back of the arms	
Displays erratic behavior – good one day , bad the next	
Craves certain foods, especially dairy and wheat products	
Problems with bowels, such as constipation and diarrhea	
Has a rapid heart rate and/or high blood pressure	
Appears bloated, especially after meals, and often complains of stomach pains	
Had body odor	
Sweats a lot	
Hands are always moist and clammy	

Left Cortex Delay/Deficiency Questionnaire

Fine motor problems (poor or slow handwriting)	
Difficulty with fine motor skills, such as buttoning a shirt	
Poor or immature hand grip when writing	
Tends to write very large for age or grade level	
Stumbles over words when fatigued	
Exhibited delay in crawling, standing, and/or walking	
Loves sports and is good at them	
Good muscle tone	
Poor drawing skills	
Difficulty learning to play music	
Likes to fix things with the hands and is interested in mechanical things	
Difficulty planning and coordinating body movements	
Doesn't seem to have many sensory issues or problems, such as sensitivity to sound	
Has good spatial awareness	
Has good sense of balance	
Eats just about anything	
Has a normal to above-average sense of taste and smell	
Likes to be hugged and held	
Does not have any oddities concerning clothing	
Has auditory processing problems	
Seems not to hear well, although hearing tests normal	
Delay in speaking was attributed to ear infections	
Gets motion sick and has other motion sickness issues	
Is not under sensitive or oversensitive to pain	
Overly happy and affectionate; loves to hug and kiss	
Frequently moody and irritable	
Loves doing new or different things but gets bored easily	
Lacks motivation	
Withdrawn and shy	
Excessively cautious, pessimistic, or negative	
Doesn't seem to get any pleasure out of life	
Socially withdrawn	
Cries easily; feelings get hurt easily	

Empathetic to other people's feelings; reads people's emotions well	
Gets embarrassed easily	
Very sensitive to what others think about him or her	
Procrastinates	
Is extremely shy, especially around strangers	
Is very good at nonverbal communications	
Is well liked by other children and teachers	
Does not have any behavioral problems in school	
Understands social rules	
Has poor self-esteem	
Hates doing homework	
Is very good at social interaction	
Makes good eye contact	
Likes to be around people and enjoys social activities, such as going to parties	
Doesn't like to go to sleepovers	
Is not good at following routines	
Can't follow multiple-step directions	
Is in touch with own feelings	
Jumps to conclusions	
Very good at big picture skills	
Is an intuitive thinker and is led by feelings	
Good at abstract "free" association	
Poor analytical skills	
Very visual; loves images and patterns	
Constantly questions why you're doing something or why rules exist	
Has poor sense of time	
Enjoys touching and feeling actual objects	
Has trouble prioritizing	
Is unlikely to read instructions before trying something new	
Is naturally creative, but needs to work hard to develop full potential	
Would rather do things instead of observe	
Uses good voice inflection when speaking	
Misreads or omits common small words	
Has difficulty saying long words	
Reads very slowly and laboriously	
Had difficulty naming colors, objects, and letters as a toddler	
Needs to hear or see concepts many times in order to learn them	
Has shown a downward trend in achievement test scores or schools performance	
Schoolwork is inconsistent	
Was a late talker	
Has difficulty pronouncing words (poor phonics)	
Had difficulty learning the alphabet, nursery rhymes, or songs when young	
Has difficulty finishing homework or finishing a conversation	
Acts before thinking and makes careless mistakes	
Daydreams a lot	
Has difficulty sequencing events in the proper order	
Often writes letters backward	
Is poor at basic math skills	

Dr. Kevin Conners, Dr. Kelly Halderman

Has poor memorization skills	
Has poor academic ability	
Has an IQ lower than expected and verbal scores are lower than nonverbal scores	
Performs poorly on verbal tests	
Needs to be told to do something several times before acting on it	
Stutters or stuttered when younger	
Is a poor speller	
Doesn't read directions well	
Gets chronic ear infection	
Prone to benign tumors or cysts	
Has taken antibiotics more than ten to fifteen times before the age of 10	
Has had tubes put in the ears	
Catches colds frequently	
No allergies	
Has a bedwetting problem	
Has or had an irregular heartbeat, such as an arrhythmia or a heart murmur	

Add up your score for RIGHT brain and compare to your score for LEFT brain. How imbalanced are you?

Dr. Kevin Conners, Dr. Kelly Halderman

How to <u>ensure</u> that your child WILL HAVE ADD, ADHD:

***Brain issues such as ADD, ADHD, PDD-NOS, Asperger's, and Autism are usually Right Cortical deficiencies therefore a relatively HYPER Left Cortex. The left brain stimulators we are exposed to in today's society exceed the right brain stimulators. Below is a brief list of things you do NOT want to do with your child as they are left brain stimulators and may contribute to such conditions listed above.

1. As an infant, get them on baby Einstein (strongly works the left frontal lobe only)
2. Get them a Leapfrog or other "learning" video game as early as possible
3. Let them play computer games, Nintendo, iPad, iPhone, texting, etc
4. Have them watch TV a couple hours a day
5. Don't let them get outside and play if at all possible
6. Don't let them run around and play make-believe as this is right brain stimulation
7. Feed them Lunchables, Sunny-D, Capri-Sun and the like

--Keep this up, be determined, and you WILL have a child with a VERY imbalanced brain and serious learning and behavioral problems!

Chapter Five

NEUROFEEDBACK

A NEW APPROACH

> "In my opinion, if any medication had demonstrated such a wide spectrum of efficacy it would be universally accepted and widely used."
>
> Frank M. Duffy, M.D.,
>
> Professor and Pediatric Neurologist at Harvard Medical School

"Never stop asking why"

For over 40 years the accepted medical treatment for neurological conditions such as anxiety, depression and ADD/ADHD has been the use of medications. Many disadvantages of this approach are widely known, such as exceedingly high cost and unwanted side effects, which ultimately lead to a decrease in quality of life instead of an improvement. Patients and families are progressively frustrated with a one-size-fits-all treatment that fails to address the actual cause of the problem and fails ask the question, "Why?" Why does a person have anxiety? Why does a child suffer from

ADHD? Dissatisfaction with the poor standard of care for managing neurological disease is ubiquitous and increasing because it is based on addressing only the "what" (a.k.a. the diagnosis), then covering up the associated symptoms with drugs. We make no forward progress when the "why" is ignored and the "what" is focused upon. Thankfully, there are other non-invasive and non-toxic ways to change the brain that identify and treat the root cause.

A new and exciting field called Neurofeedback has emerged and is gaining positive results for many people with debilitating neurological symptoms and conditions. The success of Neurofeedback is based on the fact that the brain has the ability to create new connections, in a process referred to as "Neuroplasticity." Neurofeedback sessions usually last around 30 minutes and in that time the correct pathway/brainwaves are stimulated hundreds of times. Through Neuroplasticity, the brain is essentially trained to continue to fire this desirable path/brainwave – literally changing the adverse behavior/symptoms. Neuroplasticity also allows Neurofeedback to change timing and activation patterns in many areas of the brain simultaneously. Incredibly, this leads to global improvements in attention, memory, emotional stability, and mental flexibility. This type of therapy addresses underlying causes by restoring normal brainwave functions long-term. The sole use of prescription medications to cover up symptoms can now be thought of as an out-of-date practice.

THE HISTORY

"A discovery made before its time"

Though EEG and subsequent Neurofeedback treatment doesn't tell us "why", it points to "what" and gives us a "how" to correct things.

In the 1930's, Germany was an unfriendly place for anyone with emotional issues. Experimentation in brain activity centered more around, "why one race is superior to another" and less on helping the helpless. Most doctors with any morals, including Albert Einstein and Sigmund Freud, fled Nazi control as they could see the writing on the wall. Hans Berger stayed. While he should be no one's hero, it was he who was the first to record brain waves in an epileptic patient during a seizure. His discoveries, largely on psychiatric patients at the University of Jena in Berlin, paved the way for understanding that the human brain emits signals, waves of electricity, much like a radio transmitter. These waves, energized by our thoughts, change with sensory reception and with mental focus. Berger initially found many subjects to test and compare differences in this 'radio' activity until the Nazi "social hygiene" process soon exterminated most considered mentally ill, even those in their own race. By 1941, over seventy thousand German patients had been euthanized and Berger found himself in a deeper depression than his test subjects. Whether it was from deep remorse over all he saw or his own mental illness, Berger soon ended his own life in the same sanatorium where he worked.

The great irony of Berger's life is that the brain waves he discovered are now understood to be a key in relieving the depression from which he suffered. Though he obviously couldn't realize it at the time, this electric field he measured paints a picture. Like the discovery of a new color and canvas that someone later would apply in ways, and shapes, and forms that make us stop and look and experience beauty, so Berger's crude findings allowed others to use this enlightenment to help mankind. God is peculiar that way.

Patients with Alzheimer's disease and Multiple Sclerosis show marked dysfunctional changes in brain waves. Also, those with Depression, Anxiety, and every ASD patient will show aberrancies in their brain waves. But far from what Berger and even much later brain scientist thought, the neurons are not the only brain structure conducting electricity. Glial cells also affect brain activity. Brain waves arise from a combined electrical frequency much like a crowd at a football stadium; individual conversations are silenced from the collective whole. While between plays, a noisy purr clutters in the background but as soon as the running back breaks through the defensive wall, the crowd unites in a purposeful cheer. So to your brain waves, a collection of noise from a variety of clutter becomes more organized and precise given a stimuli or intent.
We measure electrical flow, like a current; as it depolarizes a neuronal axon it must return to form a circuit. It does so by passing through glial cells surging in waves that oscillate in patterns depending on activity. This collective roar is what we measure on an EEG. When we are relaxed, brain waves whisper in a slow wave pattern; when there is activity, the waves crash upon the shore colliding together in a more haphazard pattern.

Though glial cells, specifically astrocytes, do not generate an electrical impulse, their steady electrical hum comes from discharges from the neurons. Many disorders of sleep, hypoxia, hypoglycemia, and even stroke are associated with gradual changes in glial cells ability to conduct voltage. These changes in glial function and more gross changes in neuronal conduction are what we assess in an EEG. A "Brain Map" gives us a picture of all this commotion. Though EEG and subsequent Neurofeedback treatment doesn't tell us "why", it points to "what" and gives us a "how" to correct things.

Neurofeedback is non-invasive, non-painful technique for monitoring and improving brain activity for both children and adults. As used today, Neurofeedback was developed in the 1960s, where researchers explored findings that people could become aware of their own brain electrical activity, as captured by the electroencephalogram (EEG). It was found that EEG activity could be altered deliberately by means of feedback of EEG information to the subject. Around this same timeframe, a researcher from The UCLA School of Medicine, M. Barry Sterman of was performing sleep studies on cats finding that a certain rhythmic activity was present in both the sleeping and waking state. He used this knowledge to successfully train cats to produce and sustain specific brainwave frequencies using rewards. This is noted as being the first time in history where scientific results demonstrate that behavior could be altered by EEG conditioning. Incidentally, NASA then approached Sterman regarding his work secondary to a problem they were noticing with Apollo mission astronauts. It was suspected that their exposure to continuous low levels of rocket fuel was decreasing their cognitive function. The rocket fuel was known to be capable of inducing seizures at high levels. Dr. Sterman agreed to test rocket fuel exposure on his lab animals (cats) and discovered that, the rocket fuel did indeed induce seizures. However, there was a wide variation is each cat's seizure threshold. After further investigation, it was found that those cats which had undergone the brainwave training had a significantly higher seizure threshold than the others. It was concluded that brainwave training can decrease susceptibility to neurological dysfunction. This small experiment propelled a lengthy period of research in which it was thoroughly demonstrated that seizure incidence, duration and intensity could be reduced with biofeedback via EEG training. Moving forward with this knowledge, a version of EEG biofeedback called "alpha training" became popular in the sixties and seventies, which unfortunately soured its use for serious study by most universities. And although the work of Sterman was sound and easily replicated by a number of research groups, it was never truly "picked up" for any other practical purpose other than for those with severe seizure disorder. His technique was thought to be too obscure, time-consuming and expensive by mainstream research and practitioner communities. In regards to the work of Sterman, Siegfried Othmer, Ph.D. writes:

"Perhaps most significantly, these findings---intriguing though they were---could not be fitted into a framework in which they could be understood at the time. EEG neurofeedback was therefore a glaring case of "prematurity in science," a discovery made before its time. Significant advances would be necessary in the neurosciences before the realm of EEG frequencies could be understood and integrated into the body of scientific knowledge. This is only happening now, some two to three decades later. At the time, the results remained as scientific curiosities and as such soon fell by the wayside."

Seeing its potential for further use in other conditions, researchers continued to investigate EEG biofeedback and discovered some major findings - "the observation was consistently made that hyperactivity in epileptics seemed to subside with the training. Over the years it was established that the technique could be helpful not only with hyperactivity but also with attention deficit disorder, as well as with specific learning disabilities. Just as the ADHD work grew out of epilepsy studies, these insights and findings accrue incrementally."

The Research

"...the most comprehensive form of 'integrative medicine'... clinically validated and applied."

Today, Neurofeedback is making a major come-back secondary to improved normative databases and development of technology that can properly deliver and monitor this type treatment. Neurofeedback is increasingly being utilized by forward-thinking practitioners who hear the public's cry of dissatisfaction with the standard of care and demand for alternatives to pharmaceuticals. Of the estimated two million children in the U S diagnosed with ADD/ADHD (CDC 2007), 66 % are on medication for the disorder. The medication prescribed, Methylphenidate (Ritalin) is a powerful psycho-stimulant, chemically similar to cocaine and amphetamines. Reported side effects of this FDA controlled class of medications, include problems with insufficient growth and weight and the long-term effects are still unknown. Surveys of families with children on these drugs express concern over their safety in long-term use. Yet the medical community continues to place even the youngest of children on these toxic substances is growing.

Dr. Kevin Conners, Dr. Kelly Halderman

In 2013 a Canadian research group took a look at this trend of expanding medication use for ADHD.

"We ask whether this increase in medication use was associated with improvements in emotional functioning and short- and long-run academic outcomes among children with ADHD. We find evidence of increases in emotional problems among girls, and reductions in educational attainment among boys. Our results…suggest that expanding medication use can have negative consequences given the average way these drugs are used in the community" (Currie, Stabile & Jones 2013).

The most disturbing aspect of this trend (of increased medication use) is that sound medical research clearly suggests Neurofeedback is an equally effective treatment for ADHD. This is supported by the findings of a recent study comparing Neurofeedback (NF) to placebo training in children with ADHD (Beauregard & Levesque 2006). From this study it was concluded that "NF has the capacity to functionally normalize the brain systems mediating selective attention and response inhibition in ADHD." Researchers found a normalization of brainwaves in the frontal lobes of the brain, those areas that are typically abnormal in a child or adult with ADD/ADHD. Astonishingly, they also discovered that the children undergoing NF treatment had an increase in the density of the area of the brain responsible for learning, impulse control and emotion. This means that not only does NF change the function of the abnormal parts of the brain, but it can also change the brain's structure!

"Strong research evidence also indicates that there are functional brain abnormalities associated with anxiety and panic disorder and post- traumatic stress disorder (PTSD). A particularly robust body of research has documented that depression is associated with an activation difference between the right and left prefrontal cortex.

A large number of EEG studies have established that the left frontal area is associated with more positive affect and memories, whereas the right hemisphere is more involved in negative emotion." "It would be desirable to find a treatment that also would help address the biologic aspects of mental health disorders. Neurofeedback holds promise for offering such an alternative. EEG biofeedback is an exciting, cutting-edge technology that offers an additional treatment alternative for modifying dysfunctional, biologic brain patterns that are associated with various psychiatric conditions. It has the advantage of not being as invasive as medication, transcranial magnetic stimulation, or electroconvulsive therapy, and it has been associated with few side effects or adverse reactions."

- D. Corydon Hammond, PhD, ABEN/ECNS, in his article, "Neurofeedback with anxiety and affective disorders" published, Child Adolesc Psychiatric Clin N Am, 14 (2005) 105 – 123

Another recent study on Neurofeedback comprehensively reviewed current literature on the effectiveness and specificity of NF for the treatment of ADHD. Clinically informative evidence-based data were also included in this review. Most nonrandomized controlled trials found positive results with medium-to-large effect sizes. When only randomized controlled studies are considered, the evidence for effectiveness is smaller. However, it is believed by the authors that methodological caveats, such as sample size, sample selection and the quality of the training protocol used may have contributed to decreased results. The final conclusion of this study reports, "Recent findings suggest that NF is a promising alternative for the treatment of attention-deficit/hyperactivity disorder (ADHD). Follow-up studies support long-term effects of Neurofeedback" (Moriyama TS, 2012).

In a recent paper *Update on ADHD disorder* published in *Current Opinion in Pediatrics,* Dr. Katie Campbell Daley, staff physician at the Department of Pediatrics at Harvard Medical School, reviewed the research for the treatment of ADHD. Her research concludes, "Overall these findings support the use of multi-modal treatment including medication, counseling and EEG biofeedback…with EEG biofeedback in particular providing a sustained effect even without stimulant treatment. The therapy most promising by recent clinical trials appears to be EEG biofeedback."

The results of a study by the National Institute of Mental Health on neurofeedback for A.D.H.D. were recently announced at the annual meeting of the American Academy of Child and Adolescent Psychiatry. In an interview, the study's director, Dr. L. Eugene Arnold, an emeritus professor of psychiatry at Ohio State, noted that there had been "quite a bit of improvement" in many of the children's behavior, as reported by parents and teachers. Dr. Arnold said that if the results bore out that neurofeedback was making the difference, he would seek financing for a broader study, with as many as 100 subjects."

Russell A. Barkley, a professor of psychiatry at the Medical University of South Carolina and a leading authority on attention problems, has long dismissed claims that neurofeedback can help. But Dr. Barkley says he was persuaded to take another look after Dutch scientists published an analysis of recent international studies finding significant reductions in impulsiveness and inattention.

Based on all current data, in November 2012 the American Academy of Pediatrics approved Neurofeedback as a Level 1 or "best support" treatment option for children suffering from ADHD. Although there are theories as to why it is seldom utilized by mainstream medicine, it is still a question that has remained unanswered. The editors of Child and Adolescent Psychiatric clinics of North America report, "There is a large body of scientific research documenting the effectiveness of NF for several areas of psychological or neurodevelopment difficulty. These studies have been published in numerous scientific and professional journals in the US and abroad.

Dr. Kevin Conners, Dr. Kelly Halderman

Unfortunately, many healthcare professionals are not aware of the extent of research support."

Neurofeedback has been shown to be effective, clinically for other neurological diseases such as depression, anxiety, OCD, dementia and more. The growth of studies exploring and demonstrating the utilization of NF has exploded over the past 15 years, with references in the hundreds of thousands in the Library of National Medicine. Dr. Robert Turner, MD, an expert on neurotherapy, which includes NF, says, "Now is the time, the 'coming of age,' of the field of neurotherapy, because it is now being shown to be the most comprehensive form of 'integrative medicine' mechanistically, functionally, and clinically validated and applied."

Neurofeedback can improve cognitive performance in healthy patients and those with conditions that affect working memory, attention, and executive functions such as those with major depressive disorder (MDD). Behavioral results show the effectiveness of this intervention in a variety of cerebral functions. Those with depression are able to make great improvements with a success rate of up to 90%, as demonstrated by *The Beck Depression Inventory*. Using this international standardized tool, results are not simply anecdotal but scientific.

> "Neurofeedback research has documented its value in the treatment of a variety of symptoms relevant to a brain injury population; including seizures, memory, concentration and attention, unstable mood, impulsiveness, anxiety, depression, sleep issues, and even anosmia and physical balance. Preliminary research on neurofeedback treatment of TBI is very encouraging..."
> - Neurofeedback Treatment for Traumatic Brain Injury, By: D. Corydon

Who Can Benefit

Neurofeedback allows abnormal brainwaves to be rehabilitated; in doing so this alters both the structure and function of the brain. When a normal pattern of brainwaves is restored, physiological and cognitive symptoms decline. Abnormal brainwaves often exist in those with neurological and emotional disorders, thus making NF a viable therapy for a wide array of conditions. As discussed, the current medical research supports NF for conditions for a vast array of conditions. Although no data is available to guide clinicians on the predictors of response to NF, it has been postulated that response and sensitivity to medication may be a predictor of a similar response to NF. No safety issues have emerged from clinical trials and NF seems to be well tolerated. It is important to note that Neurofeedback does not specifically target any disorder but trains abnormal brainwaves. The goal is to slowly guide the brain back into normal, healthy brainwave ranges and reconnect neural pathways that have been disconnected. The overall aim of treatment is an improvement in global brain regulation, which in turn impacts a variety of symptoms. When patients reach their treatment goals, an additional 5-10 sessions are often conducted to help set in (consolidate) the NFB training.

This is a list of conditions that are often shown in research studies to be clinically responsive to Neurofeedback:
• ADD / ADHD
• Addiction
• Anxiety
• Autism
• Bipolar Disorder
• Depression
• Chronic Fatigue
• Chronic Pain
• Epilepsy
• Fibromyalgia
• Head Injuries
• Insomnia
• Memory Loss
• Migraines
• Obsessive compulsive (OCD)
• Post-Traumatic Stress Disorder
• Sleep Disorders

It should be noted that NF may be contraindicated for those with severe learning disorders, psychotic behaviors or mental deficits. NF should only be performed by an experienced provider in those with head injury seizure, stroke, psychosis, bipolar disorder, autism, fibromyalgia and severe neurological problems. The good candidate for this therapy must be able to learn a new skill in the context of a loving, supporting environment. Those who are most successful are motivated from within and not from an external source (e.g. a demanding parent). Results from treatment can be compromised by one of more of the following: poor diet and other lifestyle choices, poor emotional support and sleep deprivation.

The Brain Map

"A MAP IS ONLY AS GOOD AS THE PERSON READING IT"

In order to create a Neurofeedback program that is specific to each patient, an initial "Brain Map" must be performed. During the mapping sessions, the captured brainwaves are used to create a visual representation for each lobe of the brain and each specific brainwave (Delta, Theta, Alpha, and Beta). This procedure is performed in a professional office-setting where a cap with electrodes is placed painlessly on the scalp. A "snapshot" of the patient's brainwaves is taken with both with eyes opened and eyes closed based upon recent research showing the changes in brain activity based on visual stimulation and sent to a normative database where a quantitative electroencephalogram (QEEG) is produced. The entire mapping process takes approximately 45 minutes. The data is then sent to a normative database where artifacts (such as eye blinks and jaw movements) are removed. The information is then processed with a large series of complex algorithms and a "Brain Map," such as depicted below (by our Brainmaster 19-channel QEEG) is produced. Problem areas are red, yellow and blue. Areas in green reveal normal brain waves.

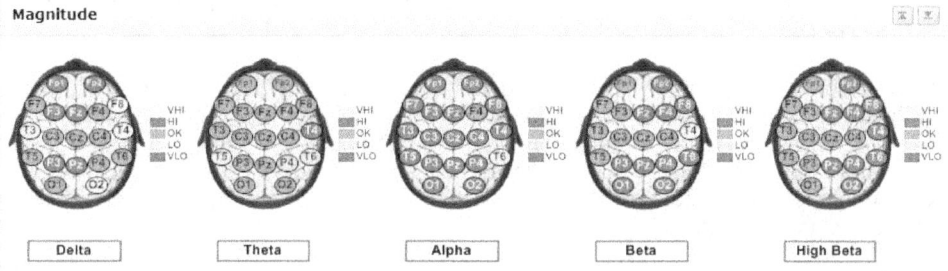

The above is an example of a MILD DYSFUNCTION (15-39 abnormal readings)

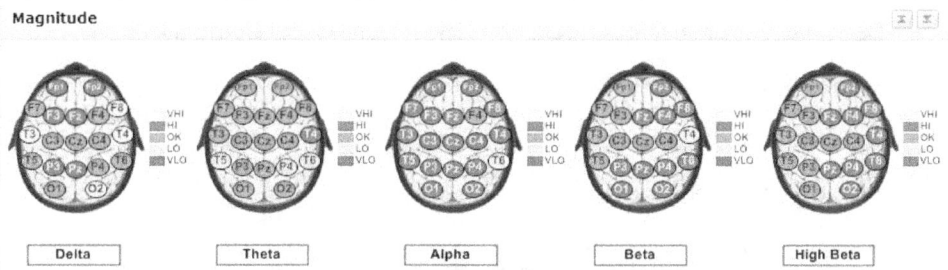

The above is an example of a MODERATE DYSFUNCTION (40-64 abnormal readings)

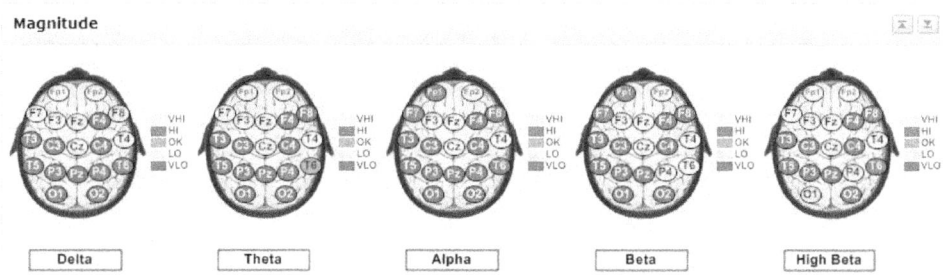

The above is an example of a SEVERE DYSFUNCTION (65+ abnormal readings)

It is important to note that Neurofeedback should be directed by and performed at the office of a skilled clinical practitioner. It is best to choose a practitioner with a strong knowledge of neurology and one who is experienced in clinical evaluation. In his book "Getting Started with Neurofeedback," John Demos writes, "A Training Plan is based on much more than a topographical brain map. It requires information from at least three clinical areas: Diagnosis, EEG data, plus an understanding or Neurology. Hence, TP = D + E + N or DEN."

The practitioner will use the "Brain Map" to identify problem areas, while combining and correlating subjective data to create a personalized Neurofeedback program. Specific areas of the brain will be targeted according to both the objective findings from the "Brain Map" and subjective from the patient's assessment. These assessments may be provided by the manufacturer of the NF device or the practitioner may use one or more of the following instruments:

- Amen questionnaire (Amen, 2001)

- Toomin's questionnaire (www.biocompresearch.org)

- ADD/ADHD behavioral checklist (Sears & Thompson, 1998)

- Beck Depression Inventory (BDI; from The Psychological Corporation)

- Burns Anxiety Inventory (BAI; Burns, 1999)

- Dissociative Experience Scales (DES; Bernstein & Putnam, 1986)

- Practitioner-designed assessments

The practitioner can also use tools such as the 10-20 system for electrode placements and the basic brain functions that are located beneath each of the electrodes (see below).

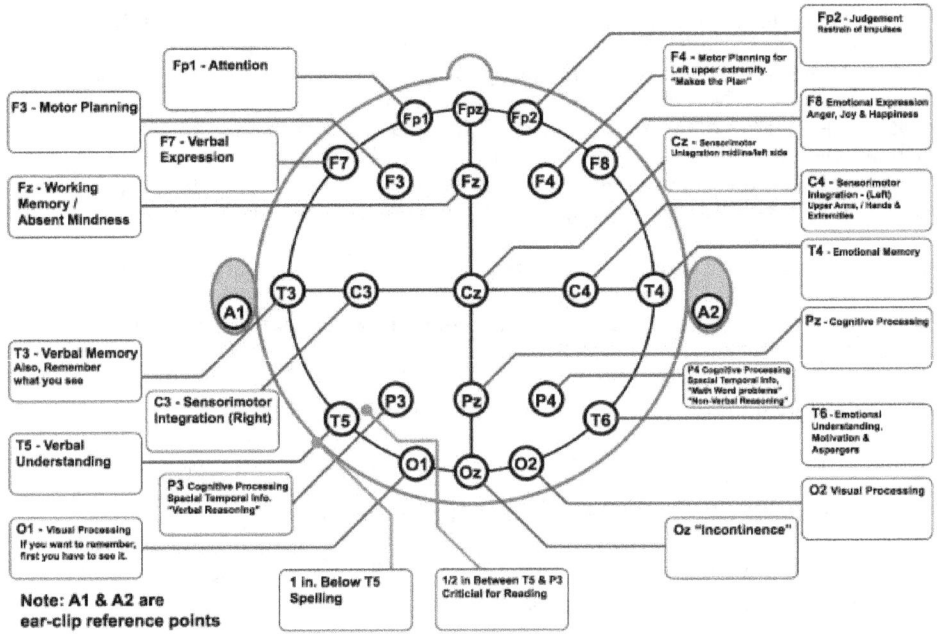

Fp2 - Judgement
Restrain of Impulses

Fp1 - Attention

F3 - Motor Planning

F7 - Verbal Expression

Fz - Working Memory / Absent Mindness

F4 = Motor Planning for Left upper extremity. "Makes the Plan"

F8 Emotional Expression Anger, Joy & Happiness

Cz = Sensorimotor Integration midline/left side

C4 = Sensorimotor Integration - (Left) Upper Arms, / Hands & Extremities

T4 - Emotional Memory

Pz - Cognitive Processing

T3 - Verbal Memory Also, Remember what you see

C3 - Sensorimotor Integration (Right)

T5 - Verbal Understanding

P3 Cognitive Processing Spacial Temporal Info. "Verbal Reasoning"

O1 - Visual Processing If you want to remember, first you have to see it.

P4 Cognitive Processing Spacial Temporal Info, "Math Word problems" "Non-Verbal Reasoning"

T6 - Emotional Understanding, Motivation & Aspergers

O2 Visual Processing

Oz "Incontinence"

Note: A1 & A2 are ear-clip reference points

1 in. Below T5 Spelling

1/2 in Between T5 & P3 Criticial for Reading

Brain waves are created by electrical impulses from neurons as they communicate within the brain and the body. The brain produces four primary types of brain waves: Beta, Alpha, Theta and Delta. Their frequencies are measured in Hertz. Beta waves (12.5-25 Hz) are primarily active during your awake-state. It is thought to be responsible for proper cognition, communication and learning. Abnormally high amounts of Beta are correlated with anxiety, OCD, over-processing, insomnia, ADHD and or headaches.

Alpha waves (8-12 Hz) are generated by the thalamus. High amplitudes of alpha waves are correlated with hyper-emotional states; low amplitudes are correlated with depressive states.

Theta waves (4-8 Hz) are generated by the limbic system and referred to as the "twilight wave." It is present briefly during the periods before you fall asleep and before you fully wake up. Low magnitudes of Theta in the posterior areas of the brain are correlated with risk for dementia. High magnitudes in the frontal areas (F3/F4) are typically present in those with ADD and represent problems with focus and attention.

The slowest brain waves in the brain are called Delta waves (1-4 Hz). They are generated by the brainstem and primarily active when you are asleep. High magnitudes of Delta (and/or Theta) can lead to brain fog. Low amounts of Delta and or Theta can be due to a deficiency of DHA.

Dr. Kevin Conners, Dr. Kelly Halderman

It is well documented that people who suffer from neurological symptoms have abnormal brain waves and therefore abnormal "Brain Maps." For example, a "Brain Map" of a person with ADD/ADHD typically has high amounts of Delta and or Theta brain waves (especially in the frontal areas), while those who suffer from anxiety have increased magnitudes of Beta brain waves. Those suffering from memory loss or early dementia have decreased posterior Theta brain waves. Neurofeedback can successfully balance and correct these abnormal brainwaves patterns, thereby diminishing or completely eradicating the symptoms of the condition.

Some general abnormal findings on "Brain Maps" include but are not limited to:

- High magnitude of Theta with low magnitude of Beta waves in those with ADD/ADHD

- Low magnitudes on Delta and or Theta can indicate a deficiency of DHA

- Low magnitude of Alpha waves is associated with depressive states

- High Alpha waves in LH compared to RH in those with depression

- High Beta waves in RH (particularly pre-frontal & parietal) compared to LH in those with anxiety, stress or bruxism

- Low magnitude of Theta waves posterior is correlated with cognitive impairment, memory loss or sleep deprivation

- The mean dominant frequency of Alpha can predict the entire speed of the brain

- Low magnitude of Beta waves in those with learning difficulties

- High magnitude of Beta waves in those with anxiety, insomnia, OCD, headaches, chronic pain

- Overall EEG slowing is associated with brain fog, slow reaction time, poor calculation, poor judgment and impulse control

- Gross posterior to anterior imbalances in Post-Traumatic Stress Disorder (PTSD)

- P3 or P5 slowing in those with dyslexia

- Increased amount of Beta at C3 C4 in those with tics

- Low Alpha in those with excess inhibitory neurotransmitter or the inhibitory areas of the brain are overactive

- High magnitude Alpha with slow Alpha dominant frequency in those with hypothyroidism

- High Delta on the left under asymmetry is correlated with cognitive problems

- High Delta on the right under asymmetry is correlated with emotional problems

- High Theta on the left is correlated with organizational problems

- High Theta on the right is correlated with impulsivity

- Slowed Alpha under dominant frequency can be associated with hypothyroidism, toxicities affecting the liver, or depression

- Increased Delta can be indicative of sensitivities to food such as gluten

The following quick guide is useful in understanding the Subcomponent Analysis system (see graphic below) of the brain mapping system (Soutar & Longo 2012).

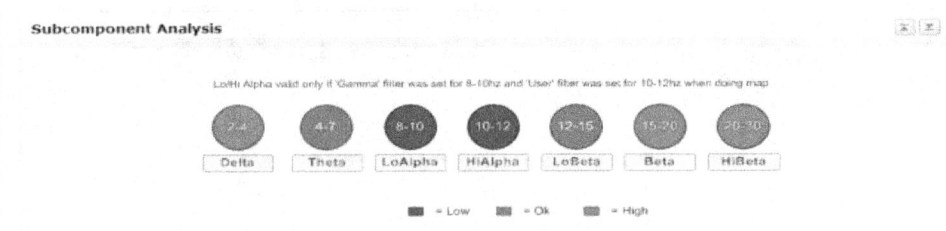

- Delta Red is indicative of white matter damage
- Delta Blue is indicative of connectivity deficiencies
- Theta Red is indicative of injury to the cortex stroke, ADD, or TBI.
- Theta Blue is indicative of lack of emotional connection of lack of memory.
- LoAlpha Red is indicative of metabolic issues, hyperthyroid or other thyroid problems.
- LoAlpha Blue is indicative of anxiety (in children it may be myelination problems).
- HiAlpha Red is indicative of possible head injury
- HiAlpha Blue is indicative of anxiety and PTSD
- LoBeta Red is indicative of anxiety and depression mixed.
- LoBeta Blue is indicative of not blocking information from motor strip, fibromyalgia, or overwhelm from sensory input.
- Beta Red is indicative of worry and insomnia
- Beta Blue is indicative of cognitive deficit
- HiBeta Red is indicative of hyper vigilance
- HiBeta Blue is indicative of under-arousal

"Brain Maps" can also provide information on the functional status of the brain, which is often necessary to gain further insight on how to successfully rehabilitate patients after concussions, cerebrovascular incidents (strokes), traumatic brain injury or anxious events. As depicted below, magnetic resonance imaging (MRI) only gives the practitioner information regarding structure.

Using Brainmaps For Assessment

- MRIs show abnormalities of brain structures.

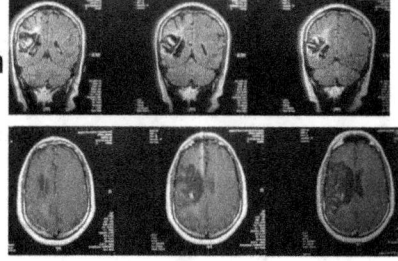

- Brainmaps show abnormalities of brain function.

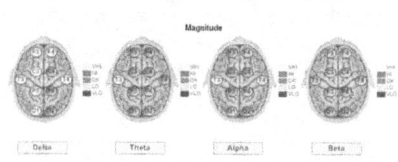

Magnitude reflection of damage due to stroke: Note Elevated Delta & Theta

NF therapy is based on the quality of the "Brain Map's" recordings. Therefore, it is of upmost importance for the patient to follow this list of instructions before the evaluation in order to get an accurate assessment:

- Alcohol should be avoided for 1-2 days before the test

- A good night's sleep is needed

- Avoid caffeine before the morning of the test

- Eat a good breakfast– avoid sugary foods

- Bring in some water to drink

- Hair must be washed the day of the test

- Hair must be dry for the test to prevent a salt bridge

- Do not use hair conditioners, sprays, gels, etc.

- All earrings will have to be removed

- Avoid over-the-counter (OTC) and supplements for 3-4 days before testing

- Report all prescription medication use

During the Session

Neurofeedback is a training to enhance self-regulatory capacity over brain activity patterns and consequently over brain mental states. During a NF session, EEG sensors are situated on the scalp. Specific brainwave activity is then detected, amplified, and recorded. The process by which a patient's brainwaves can be altered is through operant conditioning - a method where a reward is given for positive behavior. This type of conditioning was founded in the 1920's and is still widely used today in behavioral therapy, especially in the military. The operant conditioning is produced by a computer as it monitors your brainwaves while you watch a movie or listen to music.

When deviations from normal brainwave activity occur, the computer triggers the video (or music) to fade, which alerts the patient that they are outside normal ranges. In order to get the "reward" of being able to view the movie, the brain must correct its abnormal brainwave, so will adjusts itself back to a normal pattern to make the video return. For example, a child with ADHD learns to maintain low activity of the delta waves and an increase in beta waves, or the movie will not continue to play. With this, the child exercises the brain and increases his focus and attention. Within an adequate number of treatments of this process, the brain learns to stay in the normal ranges on its own without the visual reward from the computer.

Training the brain pathways and building new neural connections allows the brain to function normally on its own and symptoms from irregular brain activity, such as depression and ADHD will decline. Thus NF is a self-regulation skill that inspires growth through self-awareness. The patient also learns how to access that improved state of mind for future use outside the training session.

Some types of Neurofeedback also employ the use of brain wave entrainment (BWE), whereby brainwave patterns are modified by specific frequencies of flashing light. Using this type of light therapy can accelerate positive outcomes of NF training, as it further encourages the brain to produce the proper brainwaves.

Adding to the Success

Diaphragmatic Breathing

The brain is highly dependent on adequate amounts of both glucose and oxygen to survive. In order for NF to be highly successful, both components must be in a normal range. If oxygen or glucose is lacking, then treatment will not be at its best, as cerebral blood flow is increased during NF sessions and therefore oxygen demand will be higher in these areas. Normal breathing rates are 12-15 breaths per minute but lowering to 4-8 will likely lower tension and stress and increase total body oxygen levels. Higher oxygen levels avoid blood alkalosis, which causes arteries to constrict and inhibits blood flow to the brain.

Effective "breathe work" is key to successful neurofeedback training. More specifically, "Diaphragmatic breathing exercises" should be employed concurrently with therapy, especially in those who suffer from conditions like anxiety. The technique can be learned with no equipment in a very short amount of time.

It is done in this manner: Remove tight-fitting clothing and put on a top that shows your profile. Get a watch with a second hand. Count the number of complete breaths your take (that is, both inhale and exhale) in one minute. The optimum rate is 4-8 breaths per minute while relaxed. Breath rates of 15-25 are too fast. Next observe the way your lungs fill with air: Stand sideways in front of a mirror and take a deep breath. What moved, your chest, your abdomen, or, a combination of the two? If your chest moved most, then you are a reverse breather – sometimes known as a shallow breather. There are two factors in correct breathing: rate of breath and method of breathing. Learn to slow down your breath rate goes hand in hand with abdominal or diaphragmatic breathing. Practice the following:

- Exhale while pushing your stomach with both hands.

- Try to talk. If you can still talk, then air remains in your lungs.

- Evacuate the air until you can no longer talk.

- Inhale. You should observe that only your stomach is moving.

- Your chest should not be moving.

- Repeat (Demos, p. 58)

TAKE-AWAY FROM THE SUCCESS OF NEUROFEEDBACK

It is important to remember that NF is not a magic bullet and that in some patients the ability to "rewire" the brain may be impaired. This can also be thought of as having an inherently lower degree of neuroplasticity, which cannot reliably be predicted. Some common impairments leading to decreased outcomes are: missing a diagnosis of PTSD with an emotional component that also needs to be addressed, a less-than-accurate "Brain Map" recording or reading, a need for deep-state training or if the TP ≠ DEN. Training can also be sabotaged, as described by Demos (p.181) by:

- Motivation lacking by participant

- Dysfunctional family dynamics that over-ride successes

- Issues relating to adolescence

Dr. Kevin Conners, Dr. Kelly Halderman

- Poor cooperation, inability or unwillingness to follow instructions

- Unhealthy lifestyle practices continue allowing the inflammatory 'cause' to continue

- Critical incidents have shocked the system

Nevertheless, results can be expected when therapy is correctly devised and executed in a person with no underlying sub-clinical etiology. For example, if an underlying toxicity or a thyroid gland dysfunction is causing neurological pathology (e.g. brainwave distortion), then results will be severally diminished. The majority of patients undergoing NF training will need a complete metabolic work-up by a qualified health practitioner. Results of NF are only as good as the body is able to heal and repair and create new neural connections.

"The neurofeedback idea is intrinsically based on the findings of neurobiology," says Nikolaus Weiskopf of University College London who was part of the research team that showed its feasibility just over a decade ago. "It ties in nicely with the general trend toward biologically-based psychiatry."

Condition-Specific Information

Listed below is additional information for specific conditions from *The Clear Mind Center*. This information was gathered from aboutneurofeedback.com. Additional research and comprehensive studies can be found at the website of the International Society for Neurofeedback and Research.

CONDITIONS THAT RESPOND WELL TO NEUROFEEDBACK
ADD/ADHD

Many children and adults with ADD/ADHD are utilizing Neurofeedback. Experienced clinicians estimate that at a minimum 80-85% of these patients who complete 20-80 training sessions respond positively. Is it the most commonly treated condition because it's the easiest condition to deal with? Not really. ADD/ADHD often has many different symptoms rolled into one diagnosis which must be sorted out as part of the Neurofeedback treatment. There are some practical reasons that ADD/ADHD is the most common condition used for Neurofeedback:

- There is solid, published research on ADD/ADHD and Neurofeedback

- Increasing concerns that putting a child on medications for years is not a good thing. Parents want an alternative that works.

- For many children, medications don't work very well and have side effects that make them feel less normal, or create more problems.

Dr. Kevin Conners, Dr. Kelly Halderman

- There are thousands of Neurofeedback success stories around the country. More clinicians are adding Neurofeedback because patients are asking for it or talking about it.

Anxiety
Clinicians that use Neurofeedback report that generalized anxiety consistently responds to training and the research has proved this to be true. Significant improvements are typically estimated at 80-90% of people going through a series of training. However, results also depend very much on what other disorders may exist, meaning that we must also address the metabolic issues that surround anxiety. More complex cases that have multiple problems may take more expertise and time to respond. We still expect that these more complex cases will respond to Neurofeedback coupled with appropriate metabolic therapies. However, they take more time, expertise, and clinical skills that mean not every clinician will achieve equal results with these cases.

"In a study reported in the April 2013 Translational Psychiatry, Michelle Hampson and colleagues at Yale used neurofeedback to train participants—people who reported high levels of contamination anxiety— to modify activity in the orbitofrontal cortex (OFC), a brain area believed to play a key role in emotional regulation and to function abnormally in psychiatric symptoms like anxiety.
Two sessions in the scanner reduced their anxiety response to provocative images, and produced alterations in brain function that went well beyond the target area."
- The Promise of Neurofeedback, By Carl Sherman., July 23, 2013

Autism
Autism, PDD, and RAD are the fastest growing areas of Neurofeedback. The calming effects of Neurofeedback produce noticeable results quickly in these severely-affected populations. Due to the extreme nature of Autism, significantly more time may be needed to see results.

Bipolar Disorder
Clinical reports from psychiatrists and psychologists indicate that Neurofeedback helps patients with Bipolar Disorder become more stable and better able to reduce medications.

Chronic Pain/Fatigue
For chronic pain, Neurofeedback helps reduce pain or perhaps how the brain manages pain, even in severe cases.

Depression
Even for long-term, non-responsive depression cases, Neurofeedback typically helps alleviate symptoms. It can also help reduce the need for multiple medications, which is common for depression treatment. Depression and dysthymia are among the more common conditions Neurofeedback helps. This is not to say it's easy, clinical skills are

important and there are a variety of protocol options, depending on the comorbidities associated with the client.

> *"I've seen questions here and there on the forums about neurofeedback, and as I just finished a course of neurofeedback treatment, I wanted to briefly share my experience here for anyone considering it.*
> *It would not be an exaggeration to say that it seems like magic. I feel like a new person, or rather like an old one--my old self, who disappeared four months ago into a nightmare of panic attacks and depression. Praise God!"*
> - Blogger, katrinahopes, Neurofeedback: my experience on: March 11, 2011

Epilepsy/Seizures
Multiple peer-reviewed studies show a reduction in seizures that are non-responsive to medications and that the training effect holds. This literature is compelling in respected journals, and the clinical reports consistently reflect improvement. But for several reasons, including a lack of funding to educate physicians, the research is not well known.

Learning Disabilities
Over the last few years, two professionals in particular have published data about new brain training techniques they are using to target learning disabilities with QEEG, which was exciting news for the field of Neurofeedback. It's common for reading, math and other problems to improve with Neurofeedback and that is significantly helpful, but some clients could still have deficits after Neurofeedback training. By adding in this new technique of coherence training, a fairly sophisticated component of training, several highly-reputed professionals are reporting more consistent improvements in dyslexia, reading and math deficits, and visual and auditory processing problems.

Migraines
Therapists and doctors report that the frequency and intensity of migraines are often reduced and sometimes eliminated.

Insomnia/Sleep Disorders
The first changes clients typically observe after receiving Neurofeedback relate to sleep. This includes improvement in insomnia, bruxism, poor sleep quality, difficulty waking, frequent waking, and nightmares.

Substance Abuse/Addiction
In one published study, Neurofeedback was compared with a successful 12-step program for crack, cocaine, methamphetamine, and heroin users. Sustained abstinence was significantly greater (2 times or greater) with the group that also received Neurofeedback training. Previous published studies show similar results for alcoholics. Substance abuse is an obvious form of poor self-regulation and self-medication.

Traumatic Brain Injury
Neuropsychologists have reported that improvement with TBI often occurs even many

years after the injury and that neural plasticity still exists. Emotional and behavioral improvements are significant for this group.

The Future of Medicine

Although the Neurofeedback has been around for some time, it is now only beginning to gain the moment it well deserves, as it has been clinically proven to consistently produce results for a plethora of conditions. Advances in technology have helped NF become affordable and practical, enabling patients to have options other than the use of medication for treating illness. Wide-spread discontentment with the one-"med"-fits-all approach for treating neurological and psychiatric conditions such as anxiety, depression and ADD/ADHD has also paved the way for a new approach. Neurofeedback is safe, effective and non-invasive – it identifies and treats the root cause of symptoms, which is the future of medicine.

REFERENCES

Alvarez J, Meyer FL, Granoff DL, Lundy A. The effect of EEG biofeedback on reducing post-cancer cognitive impairment. Integr Cancer Ther. 2013 Nov;12(6):475-87.
American Academy of Pediatrics report: Evidence-based Child and Adolescent Psychosocial Interventions, released November 2012

Arns, M., de Ridder, S., Strehl, U., Breteler, M., & Coenen, A. (2009). Efficacy of neurofeedback treatment in ADHD: the effects on inattention, impulsivity and hyperactivity: a meta analysis.Clinical EEG and Neuroscience, 40(3), 180-189.

Beauregard, M. Levesque, J. Functional magnetic resonance imaging (fMRI) investigation of the effects of neurofeedback training on the neural bases of selective attention and response inhibition in children with attention-deficit/hyperactivity disorder. Appl Psychophysiol Biofeedback. 2006 Mar;31(1):3-20).

Cantor, D. & Evans, J. (2013) Clinical Neurotherapy: Application of Techniques for Treatment Waltham, MA: Academic Press.

Currie, J. Stabile, M., Jones, L. Do Stimulant Medications Improve Educational and Behavioral Outcomes for Children with ADHD? NBER Working Paper No. 19105 June 2013

Demos, J. (2005). Getting Started with Neurofeedback. New York: W.W. Norton & Company.

Duric, N., Assmus, J., Gundersen, D., & Elgen, I. (2012). Neurofeedback for the treatment of children and adolescents with ADHD: a randomized and controlled clinical trial using parental reports. BMC Psychiatry, 12(1), 107.

Escolano, C. EEG-based upper-alpha neurofeedback for cognitive enhancement in major depressive disorder: A preliminary, uncontrolled study. Conf Proc IEEE Eng Med Biol Soc. 2013 Jul;2013:6293-6.

Moriyama TS, Polanczyk G, Caye A, Banaschewski T, Brandeis D, Rohde LA. Evidence-based information on the clinical use of neurofeedback for ADHD. Neurotherapeutics. 2012 Jul;9(3):588-98.

Chapter Six

HOME Brain-Based Therapy WORKBOOK

"You have brains in your head.

You have feet in your shoes.

You can steer yourself

any direction you choose."

- Dr. Seuss

Dr. Kevin Conners, Dr. Kelly Halderman

Understanding FUNCTIONAL NEUROLOGY

We have a fascination with the brain as "mission control" of the human body. God created man and gave him a rather large frontal lobe, differentiating humans from all other species. Many of us forget that most events in our body, from the vaguest memory to muscle movement, begin with the brain. The brain is so complex that to discuss it is often overwhelming. It is the complexity, though, that is key to understanding how different areas of the brain affect different functions in the body.

This workbook is to accompany your care at our clinic. A brief, ever so simplified review may aide your understanding of WHY you are being instructed to perform the following exercises.

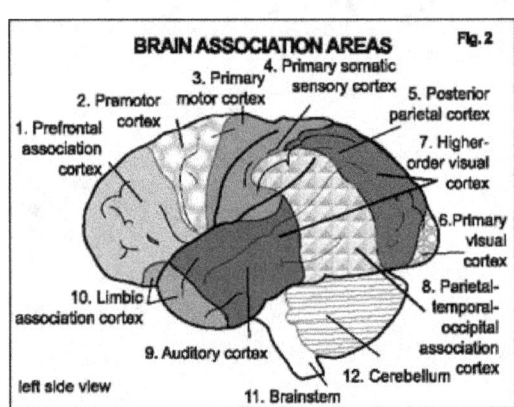

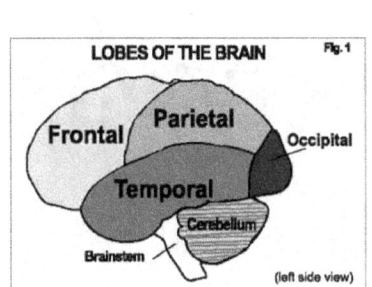

We use many terms that may be new to the average person. "Lesion" is one that sounds scary yet just means there is a problem in a particular area. When we speak of a frontal lobe lesion, we mean there is a problem with its function. Though many areas of the brain perform more than one function, here we will look to illustrate the interwoven aspects of the brain and how many areas can affect movement in everyday life. Equally important, you will learn how brain-based therapies, such as specific music, metronome timing exercises, visual stimulation, etc. can retrain the brain and help patients.

BRAIN AREAS	PRIMARY FUNCTION	SECONDARY FUNCTION
1. Prefrontal Association Cortex	Decides what we want to move	Focus, concentration, planning (a.k.a. executive functions)

2. Premotor Cortex	Decides how we should move	
3. Primary Motor Cortex	Sends signals to move muscles, initiating movement	
4. Primary Somatic Sensory Cortex	Senses muscle and joint movement (proprioception)	Helps coordinate the next muscle movement
5. Posterior Parietal Cortex	Coordinates what we expect the body to feel with what the skin, muscles and joints actually feel	
6. Primary Visual Cortex	Processes what the eye sees	
7. Higher-Order Visual Cortex	Gives meaning to what we see	
8. Parietal-Temporal-Occipital Association Cortex	Coordinates what the body feels, hears and sees	Sends information to prefrontal association cortex (1) to help plan next movement and response to your surroundings
9. Auditory Cortex	Processes language and sounds that are heard	
10. Limbic Association Cortex	Coordinates movements and other senses (smell, vision, etc.) with how we feel emotionally	Sends information to prefrontal association cortex (1) to help plan next movement and response to your surroundings.
11. Brainstem	Relay "highway" between brain, cerebellum and body	Coordinates eye movements, blood pressure, respiration,

		consciousness, digestion, bowel and bladder function and much more.
12. Cerebellum	Coordinates muscle movements	Coordinates balance, muscle rhythm and timing as well as eye movements, neck and back muscles
Basal Ganglia (not pictured)	Processes muscle movement	Processes emotions

The table shows the different areas of the brain, their primary "job," and secondary functions. The numbers on the table match those on Fig. 2, the Brain Association Areas diagram. It is important to note where the areas are, which areas are neighbors and what each area does. Some areas cross over in their involvement further establishing the interconnectedness of the brain. The act of moving a muscle is more complicated than it might seem. Generally, the process is as follows: Area #1 (Prefrontal Association Cortex) decides **what** we want to move, Area #2 (Premotor Cortex) decides **how** we should move, Area #3 (Primary Motor Cortex) **initiates** movement, Area #4 (Primary Somatic Sensory Cortex) **senses** how the movement happened. It is not just coincidence that these areas are neighbors and rely on each other.

What happens when one area starts to malfunction? The neighboring areas act as "back-up" for the primary areas. When the brain or body experiences injury, trauma or dysfunction, it tries to find a new way to accomplish the task. For better or worse, we have the ability to learn to do things right or to learn to do them wrong. When we learn to do things wrong it can result in a "miss-wiring" of the brain. This "miss-wiring" is now the brain's new "normal." The goal in brain-based rehabilitation is to retrain the brain and the body from "miswired" back to their "original wiring." Brain-based rehabilitation takes time. Just like when one learns a new language or a new instrument, it takes repetition, patience, time and effort.

Dr. Kevin Conners, Dr. Kelly Halderman

If you understand the concept of physical exercise or physical therapy, brain-based physical rehabilitation is somewhat similar. Instead of focusing only on the body, the doctor must examine function of all possible brain areas that control body movement. Once we have determined which neuropathways and brain areas are not working so well, we apply various exercises and therapies to retrain those brain areas. **The goal: as the brain "rewires" and strengthens, it can relearn how to control and coordinate brain function.** This will in turn affect overall brain function and may simultaneously address the secondary symptoms so many patients report.

Here is a chart that lists a few examples of exercises/stimulations that may be utilized for brain-based physical rehabilitation in a functional neurologist's office. Also listed are the primary brain areas being exercised/stimulated and examples of correlating physical goals.

THERAPIES	AREA OF BRAIN STIMULATED	PHYSICAL GOAL
Metronome Timing Exercises (moving a finger, hand or foot to a regular beat)	Primary sensory (4) and motor cortex (3), prefrontal association cortex (1), cerebellum (12)	Improve speed of muscle movements, decrease tremors
Auditory/Music Stimulation (specific for either right or left brain hemisphere)	Auditory cortex (9)	Improve auditory processing, general right or left hemisphere stimulation
Vestibular Spinning Chair Exercises	Cerebellum (12)	Improve balance
Joint Adjustments/Manipulations	Primary somatic sensory cortex (4), cerebellum (12)	Decrease muscle spasms, improve feedback from body to brain (proprioception)
Hemistim **(visual stimulation computer program)**	Primary visual cortex (6), parietal lobe, frontal lobe (Fig. 1), cerebellum (12)	Decrease muscle spasms, improve balance, improve coordination between eye movements and reflexive spinal (especially neck) muscles

Dr. Kevin Conners, Dr. Kelly Halderman

Example: Slow tempo non-vocal music (such as nature sounds) played in the left ear stimulates the right brain which can improve signals to muscles on the left side of the body. This is because sounds excite the auditory cortex (#9), then the parietal-temporal-occipital association cortex (#8) decides what that sound means and sends information to the prefrontal association cortex (#1) to plan your muscle movement in response to the sound. This example clarifies how a doctor might use visual (colored light) and auditory (sound) stimulation to help the brain control muscle movements and decrease muscle spasms.

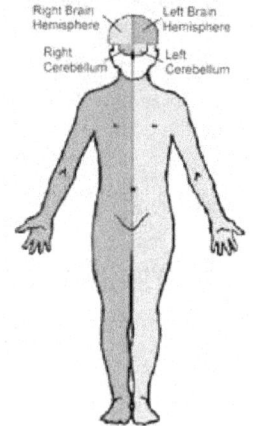

It is very important to note that these therapies are typically performed unilaterally, or only on one side of the body. This is because it is rare that both sides (hemispheres), of the brain, are malfunctioning with equal severity. In other words, one half of the brain usually has more "miswirings" than the other. This is known as **brain hemisphericity**.

Consequently, it makes good sense that all therapies must be specific to the weaker brain hemisphere with a goal of balanced right/left brain function. This is the brain hemispheric model of care. The body diagram demonstrates the general connections between the right and left sides of the body, cerebellum and brain hemispheres. For example, a stretch, adjustment or exercise using the left arm will stimulate the left cerebellum and the right brain hemisphere.

Remember, each patient has different brain "miswiring" patterns and <u>must be treated specifically as an individual</u>. This is <u>not</u> a *one-size-fits-all approach*, nor should any treatment be. Each patient's brain and body respond differently to similar therapies. Consequently, therapies need to be updated regularly to insure optimal outcomes for each individual patient.

Another major difference between physical therapies and **brain-based therapies is that brain-based rehabilitation should never push the nervous system beyond fatigue**. There is no benefit from doing twice the number of exercises prescribed and in some cases, exercising beyond the point of fatigue can be detrimental.

STOP any prescribed brain therapies IMMEDIATELY should you:

- feel dizzy
- feel suddenly tired
- feel shaky
- feel sudden body temperature changes
- feel disoriented in any way
- feel nauseous
- have any other body symptom changes while doing an exercise

The human brain has an amazing ability to adapt to constantly changing circumstances. That ability to adapt and change (plasticity) gives hope to patients with brain imbalances for it tells us there is potential to retrain those misfiring pathways Thanks to vast new brain research, we understand more about brain function than ever before. Because of this, new therapies are emerging and with them new ways toward symptom relief and restoration of muscle movements. Thanks to the brain's interconnectedness and association areas, there are many opportunities to evoke a positive change in how our brain moves our body. Brain-based physical rehabilitation is a serious option for those with neurological difficulties.

The following pages in this workbook section are meant to be used with DOCTOR PRESCRIPTION ONLY. Do NOT attempt to exceed recommendations or have others in the family use this as a guideline of any kind.

This HOME BASED program is to complement activities done in the office especially Neurofeedback based on Functional Neurological testing and Brain Map QEEG testing.

****CAUTION AGAIN: Do NOT do any of these exercises unless prescribed by your doctor!!!

CANAL THERAPY

___ to LEFT:

1. Left Horizontal Canal= Extend your LEFT arm in front with your LEFT thumb up. Fixate eyes on the LEFT thumb and rotate head to the LEFT.

2. Left Anterior Canal = Left thumb up. Fixate eyes on LEFT thumb and rotate head to the RIGHT and tilt as if you are placing LEFT ear onto LEFT shoulder.

3. Left Posterior Canal = Left thumb up. Rotate head to the LEFT and bring back as if you are placing LEFT ear towards LEFT buttocks, all while keeping your eyes fixated on thumb.

___ to RIGHT:

1. Right Horizontal Canal= Extend your RIGHT arm in front with your RIGHT thumb up. Fixate eyes on the RIGHT thumb and rotate head to the RIGHT.

2. RIGHT Anterior Canal = RIGHT thumb up. Fixate eyes on RIGHT thumb and rotate head to the LEFT and tilt as if you are placing RIGHT ear onto RIGHT shoulder.

3. RIGHT Posterior Canal = RIGHT thumb up. Rotate head to the RIGHT and bring back as if you are placing RIGHT ear towards RIGHT buttocks, all while keeping your eyes fixated on thumb.

SLOW SPIN THERAPY

___To LEFT: (for left cerebellar, right frontal lobe stimulation)

1. Spin at ¼ turn intervals (stop at each quarter turn and count to 5) to your LEFT (only do a few rotations!)

2. ADD a 'fixation point' while you perform the above holding your RIGHT arm out in front of you with your thumb up. Stare directly at your thumb while slowly rotation.

3. ADD 'non-linear, complex movement' while your LEFT arm/hand by doing the above PLUS holding your LEFT arm out in front of your and draw the "ABCs" in the air with your left hand while rotating to your left, all while fixating your eyes on your outstretched thumb.

___To RIGHT: (for right cerebellar, left frontal lobe stimulation)

1. Spin at ¼ turn intervals (stop at each quarter turn and count to 5) to your RIGHT (only do a few rotations!)

2. ADD a 'fixation point' while you perform the above holding your LEFT arm out in front of you with your thumb up. Stare directly at your thumb while slowly rotation.

3. ADD 'non-linear, complex movement' while your RIGHT arm/hand by doing the above PLUS holding your RIGHT arm out in front of your and draw the "ABCs" in the air with your RIGHT hand while rotating to your RIGHT, all while fixating your eyes on your outstretched thumb.

VIBRATION THERAPY – Place BOTH FEET on vibration device while seated.

_____ mins/day

CHI MACHINE _____ mins/day

You can purchase a chi machine at www.amazon.com

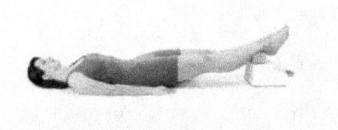

CROSSCRAWL (exaggerated "race-walk") – With eyes fixed straight ahead, simply walk (in place or moving forward) while flexing arm at the elbow as opposite knee flexes. _____ mins/day

Dr. Kevin Conners, Dr. Kelly Halderman

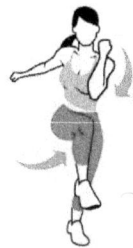

CEREBELLAR EYE PURSUITS

___for Right Cerebellar rehab (SEE HANDOUT)

1. Start at the CENTER and follow UP to the RIGHT

2. Back to CENTER

3. Then follow DOWN to LEFT

4. Back to CENTER

5. Then OVER to the LEFT

6. Repeat several times

CEREBELLAR EYE PURSUITS

___for Left Cerebellar rehab (SEE HANDOUT)

1. Start at the CENTER and follow UP to the LEFT

2. Back to CENTER

3. Then follow DOWN to RIGHT

4. Back to CENTER

5. Then OVER to the RIGHT

6. Repeat several times

Dr. Kevin Conners, Dr. Kelly Halderman

The BRIDGE POSITION THERAPY

The Bridge Position Therapy

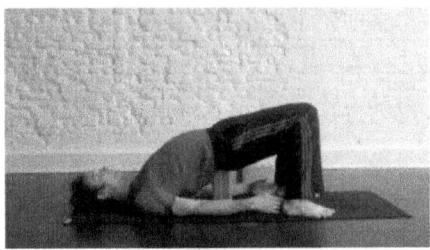

1. Start as positioned above – hold for 10 seconds

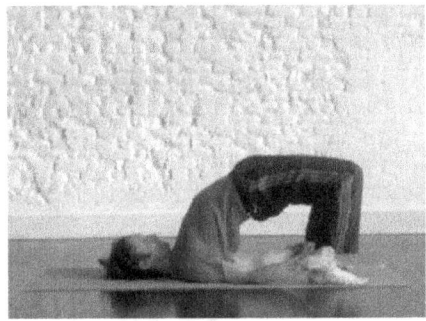

2. Move up as positioned above – hold for 10 seconds

3. REPEAT as many times as possible

PLANK POSITION THERAPY

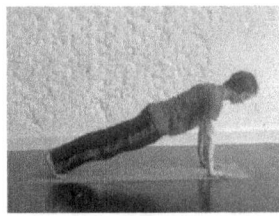

1) Start with the MIDLINE PLANK position – hold for 10 seconds

Dr. Kevin Conners, Dr. Kelly Halderman

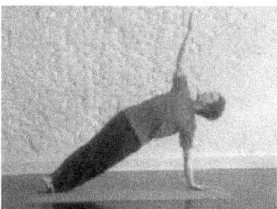

2) Move to a RIGHT SIDE PLANK position – hold for 10 seconds

3) Go back to the MIDLINE position (see #1) – hold for 10 seconds

4) Move to a LEFT SIDE PLANK position – hold for 10 seconds

5) REPEAT as many times as possible

BARREL ROLLS

1) Lie on the floor on your back

2) Make a complete roll to your LEFT (so that you end up on your back again)

3) Make a complete roll to your RIGHT (so that you end up on your back again)

4) Repeat steps 1-3 as tolerated

"GO, NO GO"

*You will need a helper to compete this activity

1) Helper snaps their fingers ONCE - patient immediately CLAPS HANDS TWICE.

2) Helper snaps their fingers TWICE - patient immediately CLAPS HANDS ONCE.

3) REPEAT SEVERAL TIMES in random patterns/order.

COMPLEX LINEAR MOVEMENT with LOWER EXTREMITY

____for RIGHT Brain Deficiencies

Write ABCs LEFT foot to the beat of the metronome. You may also simply tap your LEFT FOOT to the beat of the metronome.

____for LEFT Brain Deficiencies

Write ABCs with RIGHT foot to the beat of the metronome, music or clock. You may also simply tap your RIGHT FOOT to the beat of the metronome.

ANTI-SACCADES

___Anti-saccades for <u>RIGHT Brain Deficiencies</u>

*You will need a helper to complete this activity

1) Helper stands approx. 3 feet in front of patient

2) Helper holds a small flashlight in their LEFT hand (at patient's eye-level) and holds their RIGHT index finger at the same level about 2 feet apart.

3) Patient looks directly in to Helper's eyes.

4) Helper then flashes flashlight and then patient quickly moves eyes to the Helper's RIGHT index finger.

*Repeat several times

___Anti-saccades for <u>LEFT Brain Deficiencies</u>

*You will need a helper to complete this activity

1) Helper stands approx. 3 feet in front of patient

2) Helper holds a small flashlight in their RIGHT hand (at patient's eye-level) and holds their LEFT index finger at the same level (about 2 feet apart).

3) Patient looks directly in to Helper's eyes.

4) Helper then flashes flashlight - patient quickly moves eyes to the Helper's LEFT index finger.

*Repeat several times

UTRICLE REHAB

1) Extend Right arm out and extend thumb straight up in front of you.

2) Place Left thumb approx. 1" from your nose in the same plane as your right thumb, so that they are "lined up"

3) Focus on Left thumb, when it comes into focus move to focusing on your Right thumb.

4) Repeat step 3 (as tolerated).

SACCADES

*Home Saccade therapy can be done with:

1) OPK image on next page

Dr. Kevin Conners, Dr. Kelly Halderman

2) OR by downloading "OKN STRIPS" (left image below) at the Apple Store (on iPhone or iPad),

3) Or by going to www.youtube.com and searching for "optokinetic to the left," "optokinetic to the right", up or down as prescribed.

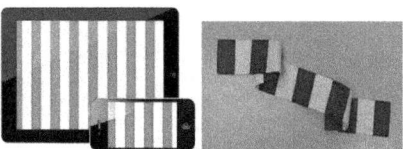

___Saccades for RIGHT Brain Deficiencies

Follow OKN/OPK strips as they move to the RIGHT.

___Saccades for LEFT Brain Deficiencies

Follow OKN/OPK strips as they move to the LEFT.

"↓UPWARD or DOWNWARD VERTICAL EYE MOVEMENTS"

___Saccades for UPWARD Brain Deficiencies

Follow OKN/OPK strips as they move to the UP.

___ Saccades for DOWNWARD Brain Deficiencies

Follow OKN/OPK strips as they move to the DOWN.

The ReBuilder®

The ReBuilder rebuilds your nerves while stimulating the brain.

The ReBuilder® treats all kinds of pain such as: restless leg syndrome, diabetic peripheral neuropathy, idiopathic neuropathy, polyneuropathy, chemo induced neuropathy, Charcot Marie-Tooth, and piriformis entrapment syndrome.

The ReBuilder® is the nerve pain treatment of choice used in cancer hospitals such as The Cancer Treatment Centers of America, the Rockefeller Cancer Center, Sloan Kettering, the Cleveland Clinic, John Hopkins, and others for their patients with chemotherapy induced peripheral neuropathy. The ReBuilder® has been proven 96% effective in a study with over 3,000 doctors treating patients who did not respond to any previous treatments.

"We refer all our cancer patients to the Rockefeller Cancer Center in Little Rock Arkansas, because they use the ReBuilder® exclusively and it not only eliminates any pain and numbness, but it can sometimes allow them to optimize the dosage of chemo and not have to limit a successful treatment regimen because of the terrible side effects. We refer our patients to them

Dr. Kevin Conners, Dr. Kelly Halderman

primarily because they use the ReBuilder. I want the best for my patients, and I hate to see them suffer needlessly." - Richard D, M.D.

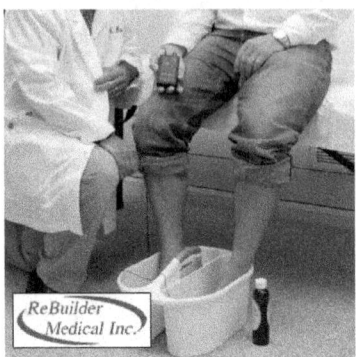

Footbath

Here is how the ReBuilder works:

When you first turn your ReBuilder on, it sets its output parameters for your physical mass by measuring the electrical analog and digital impedance of your body. It knows if it is treating a 125 lb woman or a 350 lb man. If you use the ReBuilder directly on your lower back, it knows that. You would obviously need a different amount of signal for variations like these. This is a unique safety feature of the ReBuilder. No other unit offers this level of safety.

The ReBuilder then sends out a "test" signal that represents the most common waveform for healthy peripheral nerves. (Diagram # 1) This signal goes from one foot, up the leg to the nerve roots in your back, down the other leg, to the other foot.

It then waits for an echo -like response from this initial signal. This phenomenon is similar to the patella reflex when your doctor hits just below your kneecap with a little rubber hammer and your leg kicks out.

When this initial signal reaches the other foot, an automatic response sends a signal back to the ReBuilder. (See the illustration of these signals going back and forth above.)

The ReBuilder analyzes this returned signal in a split second and analyzes for returning waveform for aberrations. (Diagram #2)

Just as a Cardiologist can take one look at the shape of the signal displayed on the EKG monitor above the patients bed in the hospital and diagnose what is wrong with the heart, we have been able to identify that the peripheral nerves have a very particular shape to its waveform, and we can diagnose the nature of the problem from analyzing that waveform. This feature is built into the ReBuilder and processed by its internal microprocessor.

Abnormalities in the shape of the waveform on the way up indicates issues with numbness; the shape of the top of the waveform indicates the ability of the nerve to deliver the signal long enough for the brain to receive it all; abnormalities in the downward slope of the waveform indicates pain, and the shape of the refractory period below the baseline (as the nerve cell repolarizes itself) indicates the ability of the nerve pathway to prepare for the next signal.

The ReBuilder then creates a compensating waveform (similar to the Bose headphones that cancel out the background noise on airplanes). Where there is too much energy displayed, the ReBuilder adapts the treating waveform to reduce that energy. Where the waveform indicates too little energy, it increases the energy in that area. This process goes on 7.83 times every second, sending a signal, analyzing the returning signal, creating a compensating signal, and sending this new signal.

The reason for the 7.83 Hz frequency is that it takes time for the nerve cell to re-polarize (or reset) itself between its transmission of nerve signals. Minerals have to squeeze through little holes in the cell wall, and then return. This takes time. We have found that if we slow down the treatment to 7.83 times per second, it gives the nerves time to re-polarize and get ready for the next signal.

A common TENS signal uses an unnatural, uncontrolled, simple signal 90 to 100 times per second precisely to stop the nerve from operating. This may temporarily give some pain relief, but can cause more numbness, and can permanently damage the nerve cell possibly resulting in permanent paralysis.

In effect, the ReBuilder acts like a pacemaker works for your heart's electrical signals. If the pacemaker does not send exactly the right signal, then the four chambers of the heart may not pump in the right order and if the signal is too fast or too slow, the heart stops. So, too, the ReBuilder's precisely controlled waveform coaxes your nerves to transmit their signals in the proper order.

Although essentially similar to TENS relative to the FDA's regulations, the ReBuilder's signals are vastly more controlled and precise.

You can think of the ReBuilder as a pacemaker for your nerves.

Dr. Kevin Conners, Dr. Kelly Halderman

Limbic System Calming Therapies

1. Remove excessive light exposure - dim lights, wear sunglasses.

2. Use rose-colored or yellow-colored sunglasses.

3. Watch less TV & spend less time on the computer.

4. Remove peripheral vision by use "blocker glasses" that have the lateral fields of vision darkened.

5. Remove excessive sound - stop all background sounds in your environment.

6. Use ear plugs or cotton balls in both (if practical) or opposite ear (of deficient brain). No I-pods!

7. Get more oxygen! Use breathing exercises such as the Diaphragmatic Breathing Exercises handout in this binder. Get out for a brisk walk.

8. Remove infections - get tested for latent infections & autoimmune conditions.

9. Avoid unnecessary chewing (gum and hard foods)

10. Do frontal lobe exercises if prescribed.

11. Do cerebellar exercises if prescribed.

12. Gargle, hum to tune as this stimulates the vagal nerve.

Chapter 7

The ULTIMATE Brain-Based Therapy

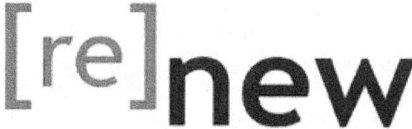

*"Do not be conformed to this world (this age),
[fashioned after and adapted to its external,
superficial customs], but be transformed (changed)
by the [entire] renewal of your mind [by its new
ideals and its new attitude], so that you may prove
[for yourselves] what is the good and acceptable and
perfect will of God, even the thing which is good and
acceptable and perfect [in His sight for you]."*
-Romans 12:2 (Amplified Version)

Dr. Kevin Conners, Dr. Kelly Halderman

Everything else in this book speaks of organic causes to brain inflammation and dysfunction. To ignore the emotional/spiritual component is to ignore the soul and, in my humble opinion, may ignore the root cause of the disorder for many. Where science argues over the differences between the mind and the brain, I maintain that there are pieces of creation beyond our understanding and things that can only be comprehended through faith.

Ultimate brain-based therapy necessitates a renewal of the mind, not just a change in the brain. Dead people still have a brain, intact with every organic neuron, glial cell and neurochemical, yet their soul is absent. Renewing the brain is useless; ask anyone with a late-stage Alzheimer parent whose body is capable of many more years yet whose mind is gone, left sadly in a soul-less-like state. There are few things more heartbreaking. This chapter is about renewing one's mind and I challenge you to read it fully even if you have different spiritual beliefs. As in everything, you may glean helpful hints to change your life.

If you think that the following is just an esoteric game – think again. What is contained in this chapter IS the most powerful brain therapy! Neurologically, as mentioned in previous chapters, there is a complicated pathway that runs from your dorsolateral prefrontal cortex (DLPC) to the midbrain (Red Nucleus), to the cerebellum (Dentate Nucleus) and back to the prefrontal cortex. It is the MOST powerful pathway to stimulate the cerebellum and the prefrontal structures and it involves one thing – THOUGHT.

What you think about is powerful. Tens of thousands of books have been written about self-talk, goals and affirmations from every perspective imaginable. It's the "secret of the ages" that is no secret at all. It is simply the way God made us – He gave us a cortico-rubro-dento-cortico pathway that reinforces ANY thoughts into stronger highways.

Let me give you an example. Should I decide (in my DLPC) that the world is a horrible place and that life is meaningless, my thoughts revolve around such a decision. My brain fires this pathway described and it becomes paved, over time, into a 2-lane highway. Pretty soon, I am a depressed person easily able to equate everything in life through the filter of the paved pathways that say 'life is horrible'. I am literally becoming a self-fulfilling prophecy.

And it gets worse. As these neural pathways regarding recurrent thought patterns mold our personality, it affects another part of our brain called the Reticular Activating System (RAS) that is responsible for alerting (waking) our brain to necessary stimuli. A good example of this might be the last time you purchased a car (let's say it was a Toyota), you subsequently notice, over the course of the next few months, all the other Toyotas driving around. Your brain was occupied about the decision of buying a Toyota so that, unconsciously, your cortico-rubro-dento-cortico pathway was firing, reinforcing your decision on such a large purchase and now your RAS takes acute notice of all the Toyotas you encounter thereby justifying the wonderful decision you made!

Put this understanding into our previous example and the person that once ruminated on the thought that the world is horrible now only sees the horrible in everything!

"People are mean, nobody cares, life's a bummer," is all this person notices as their Reticular Activating System simple 'turns-on' the brain to the pathways that have been paved.

Do you 'become your thoughts' as many self-help books proclaim? Well, maybe not, because most boys would become girls, but your thoughts are your most powerful ally or your most dangerous foe! What you think about becomes a pathway more easily traveled the more you think about it. This is the neural pathway of HABIT. When God said that sin comes from a "debased mind" (Rom 1:28) He wasn't being mean; He just knew the pathway! He also encouraged us by saying that we have a choice to, "live according to the Spirit (then you must purposefully) set your minds on the things of the Spirit." (Rom 8:5)

Even in the worst situations and the gravest conditions, even if everything in life is flying out of our control, there is one thing that we CAN control, though it takes conscious effort – our thoughts! We will ONLY, "be transformed by the renewal of your mind." (Rom 12:2) There is NO OTHER WAY!

Three Breakable Barriers

1. Addiction/Control/Co-dependency = trying to find purpose and pleasure from anything other than God's designed plan for you.

The emotional aspect of addiction manifests as a drive towards a destructive behavior that is erroneously supplying a need that can be found in or was already fulfilled with God's finished work. In earlier chapters we discussed the neural loops and chemical drives that make addictions so undeniable, but root, spiritual causes stem from unmet needs, lingering pain, and "heart holes" paved with external behaviors. I believe that brain-based therapy and Neurofeedback is essential for addictions but we must also fill the spiritual hole.

Those with 'control issues' simply subconsciously believe that exerting power OVER another brings peace. "Power-over" individuals simply squash others, many times thinking they are doing 'good'; they are 'fixing people'. I had a doctor in my office a few months back who was very ill and was seeing me as a patient. Some of his initial statement as he entered our busy office was to tell my staff what they should be doing. He pulled one aside and told her that he would 'coach her' on how to better arrange the bookcases so the 'energy was correct'. "Power-over" people have few boundaries when it comes to exerting opinion and when confronted, everyone else just "misunderstood" their intentions. Here are some telltale signs that you have put yourself in power over another though most with this problem will not be able to recognize it in themselves:

- You believe your needs are more important or you deserve to have them met before others.

- You announce what is going to happen rather than negotiate to consider the needs of others. You dictate your process rather than discuss all ideas.

- You give unsolicited advice about things not falling in your area of authority.

- You become angry and resentful if someone doesn't follow your advice or do things in a way you expect.

- You blame others when confronted or blame 'miscommunication' in order to avoid personal responsibility when hurting others.

- You view the other as incapable, pitiful, and in need of your rescuing.

- You imagine you know what is right for another without asking them.

- You think a lot of about what this person or group of people should and shouldn't do.

- There tends to be a trail of injured people behind and around you.

Co-dependency is wanting someone to do for you what you could/should do for yourself. A codependent relationship includes both a victim-player and a savior-player. Doctors, especially alternative ones, tend to develop codependent relationships with patients as they may be the only person that gives needed attention and fulfills unmet needs. This is the untold goal of all product sales. If Coca Cola can create a codependent relationship with the consumer, they meet perceived needs and produce buyers that 'cannot live without' their fix. Pharmaceutical companies thrive on codependency with ads that promise every desired feeling and apparent want.

Our office purposefully and deliberately attempts to protect both us and the patient from such relationships. Though cancer patients seemingly 'need' someone to guide and lead them through a scary and often dark time, it is our role to point them to their ONLY true hope. I am NOT anyone's savior; I am just another person occupying a destiny designed by the Creator for a specific purpose. I seek His wisdom to heal and depend on His Spirit flowing through me to accomplish anything. Patients don't need me; once they flip to needing me, I need to point them back to their Savior.

2. FEAR and JUDGMENT = the basis of man's inherited sin and what keeps us from experiencing all of God's blessings.

It is impossible, in the flesh, to live this life and *not* be tempted to judge every situation, every circumstance, everyone around us and even ourselves. It is engrained in our flesh to judge. Worse, we tend to believe that we are walking in wisdom by the way we judge people and things, when in reality we are doing nothing but creating a world of pain and conflict. We *create* the condemnation we wish to expel! The truth is that the majority of the emotional suffering you now experience is an outcome of your current set of judgments. Nothing outside of you has the power to hurt you until you place a judgment on it and this includes others as well as disease, thoughts and emotions. It is the judgment, the value we assess on anything and everything that brings us pain, depression and anxiety.

Judgment is the attachment of significance. Judgment is NOT an observation of *what* was experienced; judgment is our placement of *why*. If someone fails to repay a debt owed to me, the fact that a contract was breached is an observation; my thoughts of them 'cheating me', 'being irresponsible', 'being crooked', 'not caring' are judgments on my response to the observation of the facts as to **why** the deed was done. Making an assumption of motive is judgment and it now has power in my life based on the judgment I made.

The same is true when we judge any situation as 'good' or 'bad'. A diagnosis of cancer should inspire us to seek wisdom but we tend to judge. "What have I done to cause this? Why me? Is God angry at me? Is this a punishment?" These and other thoughts stem out of our need to cast blame; they are judgments as to 'why' instead of an observation of a fact – "I have cancer, now what am I going to do about it?" Just because it's human nature to judge and blame does not mean that doing so is in our best interest. It may seem that we throw the responsibility on someone else and even give us temporary reprieve, but ultimately we are the ones that carry the burden. Oh the pain that we would eliminate if we would just *observe* and stop judging!

I place an interesting question on my patient intake form that asks a simply question: Do you blame anyone for your current problem? Most people read into their possible answer and leave it blank but the truth is that *all of us do*, more times than we care to admit, blame someone for our current conditions. Whether we blame others, God, or ourselves, blame is a judgment rather than an observation. We can be in real physical pain and torment, suffer indescribable emotional anxiety and depression, or be dying of disease all based upon what we judge about present or past situations. Furthermore, difficult situations are always worsened when we judge the circumstance.

It may be important to define the difference between making right judgments (observations) and judging. Biblically commanded judgments do not define a reason why. They are observations that may change our subsequent action but leave the need to answer 'why' to God. This is especially difficult for people like me who have created a career of investigating *cause*. It is my job to find out why a person is sick and then administer the correct medicine. While this is appropriate in healthcare, it is pathological in life's circumstances and relationships. It may be my Biblical responsibility to observe the doctrinal integrity of whom I choose to listen to, but it is not my job to pass judgment on someone for their current beliefs.

An example was observed recently. A patient of mine spoke to me about a church that they were attending and the legalistic manipulation that was taking place. Both she and her husband wanted to leave but were confronted by the pastor who told them that their real problem was a 'spirit of rebellion against authority'. He told them that they needed to 'submit to the leaders of the church and obey the church doctrines'. One aspect that stood out in our discussion was the pastor's demands that everyone spend at least one hour each day in their 'prayer closet' and witness to one person each day. He insisted that this was Biblical as it was fulfilling the Great Commission in Matthew 28. The couple, being fairly new to the faith was confused, asking me if what he said was correct. The truth of the New Covenant is the freedom that exists in Christ. While it is true that Jesus commanded us to share His word with the world and it cannot be argued that personal communion with God is essential for our peace and growth, to manipulate people into following an agenda is flat out denial of the cross!

When we received the ability to judge good and evil we lost trust in God's goodness. When, in our innocence, we simply *knew God as good* and all He created was something for our benefit, eating from the tree of the knowledge of good and evil brought us to question God. We no longer believe God is for our good. God is 'judging us' and He finds us guilty so we judge Him and find Him untrustworthy. Ask yourself if you don't think things like this when times are tough: "I'm getting what I deserve; it's my fault, I should of, could of, ought to…" Test yourself on this; do you even have an inkling of belief that God displays His wrath through tornados, hurricanes, disasters, and the like? How many of us either thought or verbalized that the 911 disaster was God punishing America for their sins?

Here's news: God already poured out His wrath for sin on His Son two thousand years ago! Jesus became sin and took God's entire wrath, suffering the punishment once for all. Once you believed, you've been, "freed from sin, and you've become slaves of righteousness." (Romans 6:18) Believing and confessing is acknowledgment of your changed mind (repentance) about God. Those that are IN Christ are freed from the wrath of God (Romans 5:9); we are rescued through His blood (1 Thessalonians 1:10), destined for salvation (1 Thessalonians 5:9). Christ, "died for our sins," (1 Corinthians 15:3) and "He died for all, so that they who live might no longer live for themselves, but for Him who died and rose again on their behalf." (1 Corinthians 5:15)

Judgment comes through the Law and brings death. Let it come. Allow it to slay you that you may be, "released from the Law, having died to that by which we were bound, so that we serve in newness of the Spirit and not in oldness of the letter." (Romans 7:6) Let us read and repeat often, "What then shall we say to these things? If God *is* for us, who *is* against us? [32] He who did not spare His own Son, but delivered Him over for us all, how will He not also with Him freely give us all things? [33] Who will bring a charge against God's elect? God is the one who justifies; [34] who is the one who condemns? Christ Jesus is He who died, yes, rather who was raised, who is at the right hand of God, who also intercedes for us. [35] Who will separate us from the love of Christ? Will tribulation, or distress, or persecution, or famine, or nakedness, or peril, or sword?" (Romans 8:31-34)

I need to read that again, "If God *is* for us, who *is* against us?" I'll be honest, it is usually ME. My condemnation of myself and others resuscitates the Law. What was meant to kill me, revealing the need for a savior and drive me to the cross, has been allowed to live through my judgments. This should not be! But, to accept that God loves me so much that He sent His one and only Son to exchange His life for mine and die the death that I deserved is ludicrous to my human mind. This is why the Apostle John writes, "See how great a love the Father has bestowed on us, that we would be called children of God." (1 John 3:1) This Greek phrase interpreted, "how great a love" should actually be read, "how alien", or "as if from another planet" as it is altogether alien from what I know or could find in this world.

Dr. Kevin Conners, Dr. Kelly Halderman

Don't forget who you are. You are the child of the Most High God, purchased by an infinitely great sacrifice and adopted as sons and daughters of the King. Don't turn back to judgment of the Law like a dog feeding off its own vomit (2 Peter 2:22). Every time we judge we forsake the righteousness of Christ as foolish, bewitched (Galatians 3:1) souls attempting to perfect grace in the flesh. It can't be done. Jesus did it ALL. Enter into the rest that was fully won 2000 years ago to receive the power to live abundantly now.

3. Living under Condemnation = the expectation of judgment. Condemnation is a heart-sense of bad things to come… impending doom

If there is a secret to success in life, it is an open secret, available for all to know. Perhaps the most important ingredient to success is how one answers one specific question. The answer to this question governs one's attitude in both the hills and valleys of life. It sets one's perception, guides them in decisions and directs their paths. I've seen both Christians and non-Christians utilize their answer to both lead them to unspeakable joy and keep others in unbreakable despair. Our answer to this one question determines the boundaries which we live by, how big we can be and all that we can accomplish. It isn't 'spiritual' per-say and doesn't require a belief in Jesus. One's answer therefore, does not determine eternal destiny so this question may be qualified as the second most important question one must answer themselves, the first and most important question one must confront is, "What am I going to do about Jesus Christ?" However, our answer to the question below helps form the answer we will have about what to think about Jesus:

"Do you believe that God LIKES you, is the giver of only GOOD to you and desires only your GOOD?"

The religious person believes they've dealt with the most important question in life, given their heart to Christ, and yet lives under the belief that God, though He may LOVE them (since He's supposed to do that seeing that He's God and all), He doesn't actually LIKE them. Either consciously or unconsciously, they believe that God is always mad at them. They strive to accommodate God, His demands and qualifications. To the religious person, God *is* love, but He's angry at me. He expects more from me and meeting His needs to receive an eternal "at-a-boy" is exhausting. How can this be?

Religion asks, "Does He want my 'good'? Well sure," they think, "but not too good." If good things come to them they are usually balanced with a humbling event because, after all, 'God doesn't want us to get conceited'. The religious person believes that they deserve punishment and abasement and God is usually upset with them. They read of God's love and that He calls believers "His child" but then qualify His love based on their performance. God may love them because He has to; it's part of His job of being God. But really, God doesn't LIKE them. To read this in the first person is important because I think that most of us find ourselves in the "religious person" category a great deal of time.

Dr. Kevin Conners, Dr. Kelly Halderman

Let's contrast this life view with one who believes that God not only loves them but LIKES them. God only wants my good and even when difficult times come, they are but stepping stones, blessings to discover, or hurdles to strengthen me. There are no good or bad things in my life, it is all joy, and everything is a gift. God is my father but He is a good father; He invites me to snuggle up on His lap and tell me He loves me and that I am His favorite little guy in the whole wide world. He whispers sweet things in my ear and tickles my belly. He tells me of things He has in store for me and how He's planned this day as a special day with all sorts of fun challenges and treats.

> *"There is therefore now **no condemnation** for those who are in Christ Jesus."*
> -Romans 8:1

Words on which to Meditate

"Above all the grace and the gifts that Christ gives to his beloved is that of overcoming self." – Francis of Assisi

I'm sure Francis of Assisi was speaking of the 'old self' or the 'flesh' that is so difficult to overcome, that which is engrained in judgments and condemnations from Eden's inheritance. Maybe the thoughts, desires, lusts, and greed of my flesh are so difficult to put to death because we don't know what God says about the new, regenerate "I" that we've become and are in the process of becoming as truly saved believers. "Who am I," is an appropriate question. A better question may be, who does *God* say that I am? Read the following to yourself aloud:

"I am complete in Him Who is the Head of all principality and power (Colossians 2:10)." I am *complete*, no addition needed, no mixture with rules or religion, no sprinkle of philosophy or pinch of law. IN Jesus Christ, "I am alive," (Ephesians 2:5), "I am free from the law of sin and death" (Romans 8:2). Though my old self may reminisce in stray imagination I must, "put off the old man and put on the new man, which is renewed in the knowledge after the image of Him Who created me." (Colossians 3:9-10)

When the enemy whispers lies to me that in my past I once believed I remind him that, "I have the Greater One living in me; greater is He Who is in me than he who is in the world (1 John 4:4)." The world may oppress me but, "I can quench all the fiery darts of the wicked one with my shield of faith (Ephesians 6:16)," and when it tells me it has victory, I know that, "I am more than a conqueror through Him Who loves me (Romans 8:37)."

Though I sin, I repent and know that, "I am forgiven of all my sins and washed in the Blood (Ephesians 1:7)." God sees Jesus when He looks at me for, "I have received the gift of righteousness and reign as a king in life by Jesus Christ (Romans 5:17)." For I know that, "I am holy and without blame before Him in love (Ephesians 1:4; 1 Peter 1:16)," and, "I am God's child for I am born again of the incorruptible seed of the Word of God, which lives and abides forever (1 Peter 1:23)."

To meditate on the fact that HE *chose* me, even before He created the foundations of the earth is mind-blowing. He has given me, "the mind of Christ (1 Corinthians 2:16; Philippians 2:5)," and, "the peace of God that passes all understanding (Philippians 4:7)." Just say this aloud, "I am God's workmanship, created in Christ unto good works (Ephesians 2:10)," for, "I am a new creature in Christ (2 Corinthians 5:17), I am a spirit being made alive to God (Romans 6:11;1 Thessalonians 5:23), I am a believer, and the light of the Gospel shines in my mind (2 Corinthians 4:4), I am a doer of the Word and blessed in my actions (James 1:22,25)."

Think about it! God says that, "I am a joint-heir with Christ (Romans 8:17), I am more than a conqueror through Him Who loves me (Romans 8:37), I am far from oppression, and fear does not come near me (Isaiah 54:14), I am born of God, and the evil one does not touch me (1 John 5:18)."

The more ignorant I am of what God is telling me regarding WHO I AM when I am IN Christ, the more difficult it is to overcome the world. I must recite these Biblical affirmations over and over, take time to dwell on these truths and cast them as blessing over my household. For, "I have received the spirit of wisdom and revelation in the knowledge of Jesus, the eyes of my understanding being enlightened (Ephesians 1:17-18)."

Never must I speak negatively, cursing even in jest. God was not glib when He said that, "I have received the power of the Holy Spirit to lay hands on the sick and see them recover, to cast out demons, to speak with new tongues. I have power over all the power of the enemy, and nothing shall by any means harm me (Mark 16:17-18; Luke 10:17-19)." When I believe and obey His truth that I am truly a new creature, "I have given, and it is given to me; good measure, pressed down, shaken together, and running over, men give into my bosom (Luke 6:38). I have no lack for my God supplies all of my need according to His riches in glory by Christ Jesus (Philippians 4:19)."

No matter the difficulties I face, I know that, "I am an overcomer by the blood of the Lamb and the word of my testimony (Revelation 12:11), I am a partaker of His divine nature (2 Peter 1:3-4), I can do all things through Christ Jesus (Philippians 4:13), and I am an ambassador for Christ (2 Corinthians 5:20)."

In myself, I have no power, I declare myself dead, slain by the law and now resurrected by the blood, "I show forth the praises of God Who has called me out of darkness into His marvelous light (1 Peter 2:9). I am the temple of the Holy Spirit; I am not my own (1 Corinthians 6:19). I am the head and not the tail; I am above only and not beneath (Deuteronomy 28:13). I am His elect, full of mercy, kindness, humility, and longsuffering (Romans 8:33; Colossians 3:12). I am delivered from the power of darkness and translated into God's kingdom (Colossians 1:13)."

"I am redeemed from the curse of sin, sickness, and poverty (Deuteronomy 28:15-68; Galatians 3:13), firmly rooted, built up, established in my faith and overflowing with gratitude (Colossians 2:7). I speak boldly because, "I am called of God to be the voice of His praise (Psalm 66:8; 2 Timothy 1:9)."

I will NEVER give up and never give in for I know that, "I am healed by the stripes of Jesus (Isaiah 53:5; 1 Peter 2:24), I am raised up with Christ and seated in heavenly places (Ephesians 2:6; Colossians 2:12), I am greatly loved by God (Romans 1:7; Ephesians 2:4; Colossians 3:12; 1 Thessalonians 1:4), and I am strengthened with all might according to His glorious power (Colossians 1:11)."

Victory over my flesh, this world and the enemy is secure and complete when, "I am submitted to God, and the devil flees from me because I resist him in the Name of Jesus (James 4:7). For God has not given us a spirit of fear; but of power, love, and a sound mind (2 Timothy 1:7). For this reason, I press on toward the goal to win the prize to which God in Christ Jesus is calling us upward (Philippians 3:14)."

Dear Lord, may I always keep firmly at the forefront of my mind the unshakeable, unchangeable fact that, "It is not I who live, but Christ lives in me (Galatians 2:20)."

Daily Practice

Biblical Truths to "Practice Believing". We are called to "put off the old self" and "put on Christ" (Ephesians 4:22-23) which means to literally remove false beliefs we have of ourselves, others and God and be brainwashed in the truth of who God says we are and who He says that He is. Below are some verses to read daily. Meditate on them. Let the truth hit you hard for you are a prized possession of the Most High King.

Nothing you could ever do or have ever done could make God love you any more or any less than He already does. He chose you before the foundations of the earth were set to be His son/daughter and you are perfect in His sight. Crawl up on His lap and recite these verses to yourself constantly. Imagine Him stroking your hair and whispering, "I love you my precious child," in your ear.

Who I Am In Christ AFFIRMATIONS:

I AM GOD'S...

· Possession! I am His and that can never change. - Genesis 17:8/ 1Cor 6:20

· Child. Nothing I ever do or don't do will change this fact! - John 1:12

· Workmanship. He molds and shapes me to the image of His Son! - Ephesians 2:10

· Friend. HE chooses to call me 'friend'. - James 2:23

· Temple. HE dwells inside me through His Holy Spirit. - 1 Corinthians 3:16/ 6:16

Dr. Kevin Conners, Dr. Kelly Halderman

· Vessel. Though cracked and broken, the contents in me are precious. - 2 Timothy 2:2

· Co-laborer. I work not to please God but to know Him more deeply and to learn how to REST in Him - 1 Timothy 5:18

· Witness. As I simply allow His Spirit to shine through me, not by my works but by yielding to Him. - Acts 1:8

· Soldier. I submit to His authority. - 2 Timothy 2:3

· Ambassador. I am a co-bearer of God on earth. - 2 Corinthians 5:20

· Building. I am His personal creation that He planned before He even created the earth. - 1 Corinthians 3:9

· Husbandry. (His valued possession) - 1 Corinthians 3:9

· Minister/instrument. Acts 26:16 / 1 Timothy 4:6

· Chosen. He picked me because He LIKES me. - Ephesians 1:4

· Beloved. I intimately cuddle with my Daddy. - Romans 1:7/ 2 Thessalonians 2:13

· Precious jewel. He tells me this every day. - Malachi 3:17

· Heritage. I am His namesake whom He is so proud of. - 1 Peter 5:3

I HAVE BEEN...

· Redeemed by the blood. It is NOT by my good deeds that makes Him love me more nor can the bad things I've done make Him love me any less. It is impossible for Him to do either because He MADE me His child because of what HE already did through His Son. It's a 'done deal'!!! - Revelation 5:9

· Set free from sin /condemnation. Because of Him I expect ONLY GOOD in my life today. I no longer condemn myself or am condemned by others. Impending doom has ALL disappeared. Only goodness and mercy awaits me every morning and they are new each day!!! - Romans 8:1-2

· Set free from Satan's control. The ONLY power over me is my own choices now and I choose FREEDOM in Christ with ALL the rewards of EVERY promise! - Colossians 1:13

· Chosen before foundation of world. I am hand-picked to be on the winning team. - Ephesians 1:4

· Predestined to be like Jesus. God sees ONLY Jesus when He looks at me. I am white as snow and pure in His eyes. He smiles at me. - Ephesians 1:11

· Forgiven of all my trespasses. What Jesus did 2000 years ago was done once and for all. He paid the price for me. I simply believe and receive the free gift. Thanks you! - Colossians 2:13

Dr. Kevin Conners, Dr. Kelly Halderman

· Washed in the blood of the Lamb. I am cleansed. Let me learn to rest in Him and be filled with His Spirit so I may reveal the fruits to everyone I meet. - Revelation 1:5

· Given a sound mind. I claim this for peace in difficult times. - 2 Timothy 1:7

· Given the Holy Spirit. I quiet my mind and emotions to simply find comfort in the fact that God placed His Spirit inside of me. - 2 Corinthians 1:22

· Adopted into God's family. Natural babies enter into a family and parents don't get to 'send them back' but adopted children were chosen, knowing the faults and weaknesses. God picked me while I was still a sinner, dirty and an enemy of His. He STILL picked me because His love for me exceeded my sins against Him. - Romans 8:15

· Justified freely by his grace. I have been made just, forgiven, purified, and given mercy because that's just who God IS. It had nothing inherently to do with me, it was a free gift. My right-standing before God is all because of what HE has done and needs only my acceptance. - Romans 3:24

· Given all things pertaining to life. Religion strives after God; God says, "Stop, I'm already here and have already made a way." - 2 Peter 1:3

· Given great and precious promises. ALL the promises of God are YES in Jesus for me! - 2 Peter 1:4

· Given ministry of reconciliation. I can only give what I have to give. To the degree that I receive God's mercies (new and available every day for me) is the proportion that I can give them to others. - 2 Corinthians 1:22

· Authority over the power of enemy. There is NO more fear of ANY enemy!!! - Luke 10:19

· Access to God. I now freely come before His throne knowing all I ask in His name is already mine in Christ Jesus. - Ephesians 3:12

· Been given wisdom. This is what we are to FIRST ask for in every seemingly troubled time. He freely gives me wisdom and I NEVER doubt for I am a single-minded man and stable in all my ways! -Ephesians 1:8, James

I AM...

· Complete in him. There is nothing I add but my surrender to Him. - Colossians 2:10

· Free forever from sin's power. Though I 'mess-up' and choose wrong paths often, forgivness has already been granted and His mercy is new again today. - Romans 6:14

· Sanctified. He daily changes me, teaches me, and reminds me that He is good and wants only my best. -1 Corinthians 6:11

· For the Master's use. He plans my ways and ordains my day. I quietly listen to His leading and learn to obey His quiet whispers. - 2 Timothy 2:21

Dr. Kevin Conners, Dr. Kelly Halderman

· Loved eternally. Nothing could ever separate me from His love! - 1 Peter 1:5 /

· Eternally kept in the palm of his hand. - John 10:29

· Kept from falling. He always provides safe passage through any storm. - Jude 1:24

· Kept by the power of God. His strength is always at my disposal. - 1 Peter 1:5

· Not condemned. Today brings more blessings. Though often disguised as struggles, God turns all things, even problems, to good for me. - Romans 8:1-2

· One with the Lord. I am bound, chained, sealed and tattooed with His personal guarantee! - 1 Corinthians 6:17

· On my way to heaven. I am always looking at everything with an eternal perspective. - John 14:6

· Quickened by his mighty power. My ears are tuned to His calling. - Ephesians 2:1

· Seated in heavenly places. Even when my day seems so hard, I am keep focusing on facts. Facts like: the spiritual realm is more real than the physical; the victory over this situation has already been established; and healing is already mine in my spirit – all comfort me. - Ephesians 1:3

· The head and not the tail. God has set me in high places – not because of my holiness but because of His. - Deuteronomy 28:13

· Light in the darkness. I lay down my rights, my will, and my flesh to let the Spirit shine through me. His light is the brightest in the darkest of times. - Matthew 5:14

· Candle in a dark place. Candles have the unique ability to light other's candles. This I choose to do – be a light to others! - Matthew 5:15

· City set on a hill. His love can no longer be hidden in me; I make it evident to all. I have perfect peace where there is no peace, love where it is not deserved, patience where it is not earned, joy through sadness, kindness to the grumpy, and show God's goodness in perfect self-control. - Matthew 5:14, Galatians

· Salt of the earth. Salt preserves; it protects and keeps fresh. I am the salt to all I meet. - Matthew 5:13

· His sheep. Sheep are valuable commodities. I am the sign of God's riches. - Psalms 23 / Psalms 100:3/ John 10:14

· A citizen of heaven. I have the rights of full citizenship in Heaven with all its rights and rewards. - 1 Peter 2:11

· Hidden with Christ in God. The ease of life is found when I am fully yoked with Him. He then carries my burdens. - Psalms 32:7

· Protected from the evil one. No troubles will again overtake me; victory is always secure. - 1 John 5:18

· Kept by the power of God. It is HIS might and strength in which I depend. I hold His hand and He gives me victory. - 1 Peter 1:5

· Secure in Christ. There is surety in Him; I am safe. He will never let me go! - John 10:28-29

· Set on a Rock. My foundation is solid; I can stand tall; I am immovable and unshakable. - Psalms 40:2

· More-than-a-conqueror. I'm not just an overcomer, I'm victorious. All that I put my hand to is successful. - Romans 8:37

· Born again. I am made completely new. This was not just an event in my past but a present reality. His mercies are fresh for the taking every day. - 1 Peter 1:23

· A victor. I share the spoils of victory – every joy, abundance, and supply that I'll ever need and always given more than enough! - 1 John 5:4

· Healed by his strips. Jesus died for my healing; it's a done-deal. Though we all will die, my spirit is completely healed and I choose to walk as and live like a healed, healthy and whole person right now! - Isaiah 53:6

· Covered by blood of Jesus. What God did needs no addition and cannot be improved upon. Every area of my life, my deeds and thoughts are covered by the redemptive power of Christ. - Revelation 12:11, 1 Peter 1:19

· Sheltered under his wing. He is my protector; He stands in front of me in a battle and carries me when I tire. - Psalms 91:4

· Hidden in secret place of the Almighty. I now labor only to enter into His rest. - Psalms 91:1

I HAVE...

· Access to the Father. Daily I come before Him to receive His grace. - Romans 5:2

· A home in heaven waiting for me. I will be completely perfected. - John 14:1-2

· All things in Christ. All His promises are 'yes'. - 2 Corinthians 5:17

· A living hope. God's hope never fails and never disappoints. - 1 Peter 1:3

· An anchor to my soul. His anchor holds me back from running off into trouble, trying to please Him doing some religious thing, and falling into my own foolishness. - Hebrews 6:19

· A hope that is sure and steadfast. He never fails! - Hebrews 6:19

· Authority to tread on serpents. Though I go through seasons of trouble - Nothing in this world will have victory over me. - Luke 10:19

· Power to witness. My life will be my greatest witness. - Acts 1:8

· The tongue of the learned. I rely on and freely receive God's wisdom. - Isaiah 50:4

· The mind of Christ. I am daily, more-greatly perfected. 1 Corinthians 2:16

· Peace with God. He LIKES me, is NEVER mad at me, always takes joy in me and even when I sin He gently beckons me home. - Romans 5:1

· Faith as a grain of mustard seed is more than enough to trust God in everything! - Luke 17:6

I CAN...

· Do all things through Christ. He IS my strength. - Philippians 4:13

· Find mercy and grace to help in all situations. - Hebrews 4:16

· Come boldly to the throne of grace. I can bring every request for He is MY daddy! - Hebrews 4:16

· Quench all the fiery darts of every day's problems. - Ephesians 6:16

· Declare liberty to captives. I am FREE from the Law that did its work in me. It drove me to the undeniable need for a merciful Savior. Isaiah 61:1

· Pray always and everywhere. Prayer is talking to God and I quiet my mind to listen to Him. Like all His sheep, I hear His voice. - Luke 21:36

I CANNOT...

· Be separated from God's love. It is impossible for Him to love me either more or less; His love never fails! - Romans 8:35-39

· Perish or be lost. He is my everlasting fortress. I am adopted into His family and am now a full child with all the inheritances that belong to Christ. - John 10:28, John 3:16

· Be taken out of my Father's hand. Nothing, in this world or the next, can pluck me from my Father's hand. - John 10:29

· Be charged or accused. There is NO more condemnation for me. When I feel doubt or impending doom I now say, "This no longer serves me or has power over me, for there is now therefore NO condemnation for those who are in Christ!" - Romans 8:33, 1 Corinthians 11:32

Dr. Kevin Conners, Dr. Kelly Halderman

Dr. Kevin Conners, Dr. Kelly Halderman

Other Sources to explore:

- Begley, S. (1996, February 19). Your child's brain. Newsweek, 127, 55-62.
- Berk, L. (1994). Infants and children: Prenatal through early childhood. Boston, MA: Allyn and Bacon.
- Carnegie Corporation of New York. (1994). Starting points for young children. New York: Carnegie Corporation of New York.
- Jabs, C. (1996, November). Your baby's brainpower. Working Mother, 19, 24-28.
- Nash, J. (1997, February 3). Fertile minds. Time, 149, 48-56.
- Alivisatos, A. P. et al. Science 339, 1284–1285 (2013).
- Kettenmann, H. & Ransom, B. R. (eds) Neuroglia 3rd edn (Oxford Univ. Press, 2013).
- Fields, R. D. The Other Brain (Simon & Schuster, 2009).
- Alivisatos, A. P. et al. Neuron 74, 970–974 (2012).
- Schafer, D. P. et al. Neuron 74, 691–705 (2012).
- Fields, R. D. et al. The Neuroscientist.
- The Role of the ω-3 Fatty Acid DHA in the Human Life Cycle, Sarah J. Carlson, MD, MSc, Erica M. Fallon, MD, Brian T. Kalish, Kathleen M. Gura, Mark Puder, MD, JPEN J Parenter Enteral Nutr January 2013 vol. 37 no. 1 15-22
- Chronic prenatal exposure to the 900 megahertz electromagnetic field induces pyramidal cell loss in the hippocampus of newborn rats, O Bas, Department of Anatomy, Rize University School of Medicine, Rize, Turkey
- Fetal alcohol spectrum disorders: Fact sheet. Centers for Disease Control and Prevention. http://www.cdc.gov/ncbddd/fasd/documents/FASD_english_spanish.pdf. Accessed March 30, 2011.
- Bailey BA, et al. Pregnancy and alcohol use: Evidence and recommendations for prenatal care. Clinical Obstetrics and Gynecology. 2008;51:436.
- Effects of alcohol on a fetus. Substance Abuse and Mental Health Services Administration. http://store.samhsa.gov/shin/content//SMA07-4255/SMA07-4255.pdf. Accessed March 30, 2011.
- Wake, H. Lee, P. R. & Fields, R. D. Science 333, 1647–1651 (2011).
- Neuropsychological development of behavior attributed to frontal lobe functioning in children, Developmental Neuropsychology, Volume 1, Issue 4, 1985, Passler
- Zatorre, R., Fields, R. D. & Johansen-Berg, H. Nature Neurosci. 15, 528–536 (2012).
- Han, X. et al. Cell Stem Cell 12, 342–353 (2013).
- Neuroscience: Solving the brain 17 July 2013
- The benefits of brain mapping 17 July 2013
- Whole human brain mapped in 3D 20 June 2013
- Behind the scenes of a brain-mapping moon shot 06 March 2013
- Was Hitler right to invade Russia in 1941? by Andrew Wright
- Limbic abnormalities in affective processing by criminal psychopaths as revealed by functional magnetic resonance imaging, Biological Psychiatry, Volume 50, Issue 9, 1 November 2001, Pages 677–684

Dr. Kevin Conners, Dr. Kelly Halderman

- Abnormalities in emotion processing within cortical and subcortical regions in criminal psychopaths: evidence from a functional magnetic resonance imaging study using pictures with emotional content, Biological Psychiatry, Volume 54, Issue 2, 15 July 2003, Pages 152–162
- Our brains shrinking, The Courier-Mail, 7 February 2011, p. 21.
- Santini, J., Are brains shrinking to make us smarter?, The Sydney Morning Herald, news.smh.com.au, 6 February 2011. Return to text.
- E.g. Milford Wolpoff, also at the University of Michigan.
- Woodmorappe, J., How different is the cranial-vault thickness of Homo erectus from modern man? J. Creation 14(1):10–13, 2000; creation.com/cranium.
- Probiotics treatment improves diabetes-induced impairment of synaptic activity and cognitive function: Behavioral and electrophysiological proofs for microbiome–gut–brain axis, S. Davaria, S.A. Talaeib, H. Alaeia, M. salami
- Neurofeedback helps relieve chemo brain symptoms, Cleveland researcher finds, Angela Townsend, The Plain Dealer, April 22, 2013
- Neuroplasticity: Your Brain's Amazing Ability to Form New Habits, Mike Torres http://www.refocuser.com/2009/05/neuroplasticity-your-brains-amazing-ability-to-form-new-habits/#sthash.eAKpD70N.dpuf
- The Mind and the Brain: Neuroplasticity and the Power of Mental Force Paperback, by Jeffrey M. Schwartz (Author) , Sharon Begley
- The Neuroscience of Observing Consciousness & Mirror Neurons in Therapeutic Hypnosis, American Journal of Clinical Hypnosis, Volume 48, Issue 4, 2006
- Gluten Sensitivity and the Impact on the Brain, Dr. David Perlmutter, MD
- Cytokines, inflammation, and brain injury: role of tumor necrosis factor-alpha, Cerebrovasc Brain Metab Rev. 1994 Winter;6(4):341-60.
- Consequences of Repeated Blood-Brain Barrier Disruption in Football Players, Nicola Marchi equal contributor, Jeffrey J. Bazarian equal contributor, Vikram Puvenna, Mattia Janigro, Chaitali Ghosh, Jianhui Zhong, Tong Zhu, Eric Blackman, Desiree Stewart, Jasmina Ellis, Robert Butler, Damir Janigro

Further Research:

Doing Neurofeedback, A Condensed and Comprehensive Guide to the Practice of NFB
Dr. Richard Soutar, PhD
Published by the author, updated 2007

Getting Started with Neurofeedback
(an introduction to theory and practice – useful reference for clinical approaches) John N. Demos
Norton (2005)

Awakening the Mind – A Guide to Mastering the Power of Your Brain Waves
(hands-on tips for self-mastery; useful meditations and imagery for use with patients) Anna Wise
Tarcher-Penguin (2002)

Dr. Kevin Conners, Dr. Kelly Halderman

A Symphony in the Brain – The Evolution of The New Brain Wave Biofeedback (must have to understand history of the development of NFB; part of the story) Jim Robbins
Grove Press (2000)

A Guide to Neurofeedback
(great reference handbook-excellent neuroanatomy diagrams, clinical applications) Thompson & Thompson
Published by The Association for Applied Psychophysiology and Biofeedback (2003)

Handbook of Neurofeedback – Dynamics and Clinical Applications
(theoretical, but excellent resource with cited references) James R. Evans, PhD
Haworth Medical Press (2007)

Change Your Brain, Change Your Life
The Breakthrough Program for Conquering Anxiety, Depression, Obsessiveness, Anger and Impulsiveness
Daniel G. Amen, MD
Three Rivers Press, NY (2004)

Power Up Your Brain
(Dr. Perlmutter is a solid reference for nutritional concerns; discusses the spiritual side of brain fitness)
The NeuroScience of Enlightenment
Dr. David Perlmutter & Alberto Villoldo
Hay House (2011)

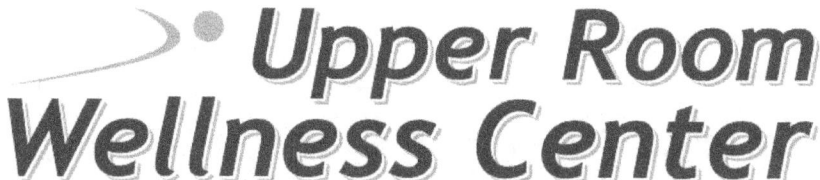

Thyroid - ADD/ADHD - Depression/Anxiety - Autoimmune - Infertility

www.UpperRoomWellness.com

651.739.1248

www.ingramcontent.com/pod-product-compliance
Lightning Source LLC
Chambersburg PA
CBHW060454290526
45791CB00001B/120